ASPECTS OF SOCIAL AND ECONOMIC HISTORY

The Story of Medicine

by R. K. Allday, M.B., B.S.

GINN AND COMPANY LTD
18 BEDFORD ROW, LONDON W.C.1.

ACKNOWLEDGEMENTS

We acknowledge with thanks the gracious permission of Her Majesty the Queen to reproduce the illustration on p. 31, in the Royal Library, Windsor Castle.

We are grateful to the following for permission to use copyright material as follows; the drawings on pp. 7 and 25 are by Pamela Mara:
R. K. Allday (frontispiece, pp. 45, 55, 85, 108 and facing p. 33); *The Architectural Review* (p. 104); Barnaby's Picture Library (pp. 21 and 93); the Cambridge Instrument Co. Ltd. (p. 42); Department of Medical Illustration, the Royal Postgraduate Medical School, Hammersmith Hospital (p. 38); Encyclopédie par l'Image Pasteur, photo Hachette (facing p. 49); D. Guthrie, *The History of Medicine*, published by T. Nelson and Sons Ltd. (p. 71); *Illustrated London News* (p. 96, top illustration); C. Kerenyi, *Askelepios*, published by Thames and Hudson Ltd. (p. 14); The Keystone Press Agency Ltd. (p. 66); Laignel-Lavastine, *Histoire Générale de la Médicine* published by Albin Michel, Paris (p. 58); *Medical News* (p. 70); the Ministry of Health (p. 86); Musee Conde a Chantilly (p. 30); Oxford University Press, New York (p. 9); the National Museum, Copenhagen (p. 6); Pace Photographic Agency (p. 107); La Réunion des Musées Nationaux (p. 81); The Council of the Royal College of Surgeons of England (facing p. 65); Royal College of Surgeons, Edinburgh (p. 79); C. Singer and E. A. Underwood, *A Short History of Medicine*, published by The Clarendon Press, Oxford (pp. 44, 35, 51, 59, 72, 96, lower illustration); The Staples Press (p. 64); J. Thorwald, *Science and Secrets of Early Medicine*, published by Thames and Hudson (pp. 7, 11 and 12) the Trustees of the British Museum (pp. 20 and 91); the Wellcome Institute of the History of Medicine (pp. 25, 28, 35, lower illustration, 40, 47, 50, 67, 78, 87, 101 and facing pp. 16, 17, 48 and 64); the Witt Library, the Courtauld Institute of Art (p. 90).

GI NN

 106903 SBN 6022 1263 4
Phototypeset by Oliver Burridge Filmsetting Limited, Crawley, Sussex
Printed in Gt. Britain at the Pitman Press, Bath

CONTENTS

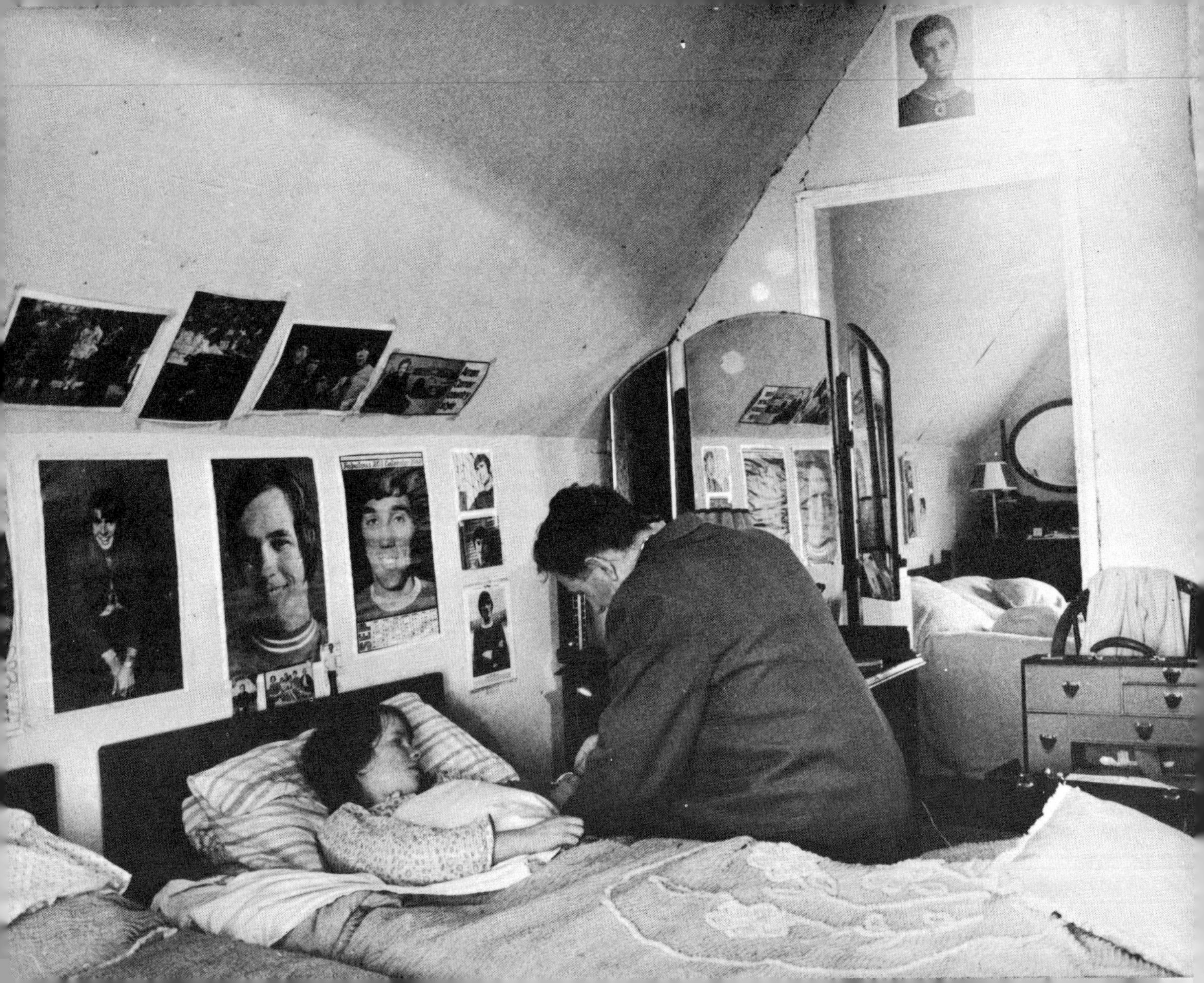

CHAPTER ONE
Prehistoric medicine

Ever since man has lived on this earth there must have been accident and injury, illness and disease, and there must have been attempts to help those who were injured or ill. The story of medicine is the story of how men have attempted to deal with the problems of illness and injury over the years.

There is much that we do not know of the past, much that never will be known, but every year archaeologists and others, searching in the relics of the past, uncover further information of how men lived.

Records, in the form of words and pictures carved in stone, go back something like five thousand years. Of these we shall see more, particularly when we look at ancient Egypt. But the practice of medicine began long before these records were made and, although there are no written records to tell of it, there is evidence to show that even major operations took place.

When a man dies, whether he is buried or not, the soft parts of the body gradually disappear but the bones do not. The bones are likely to remain, often for many thousands of years, and from these archaeologists have discovered evidence of prehistoric surgery.

In many parts of the world including Britain bones, sometimes whole skeletons, have been found, showing evidence of injury and disease. Bones that have healed after being broken have sometimes been so well in place as to suggest that the limb had been splinted and the patient nursed.

The most interesting finds, however, have been skulls from men who lived at least as long ago as the Stone Age, which have evidence of surgical operations on them. Hundreds of skulls, in many different parts of the world, have now been discovered on which the operation of trephining had been performed.

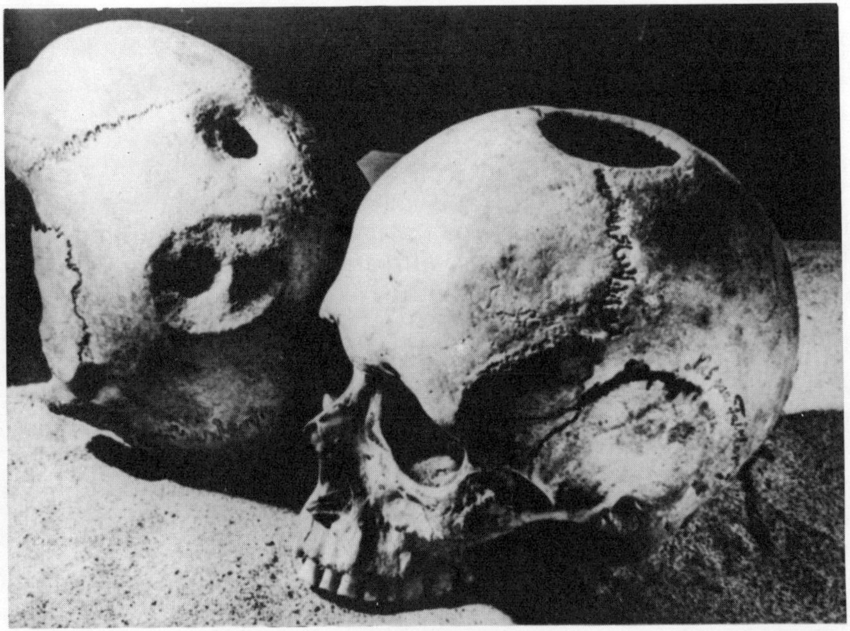

Prehistoric skulls clearly showing new bone growth (healing) after trephination

This operation consists of removing a piece of bone from the surface of the skull. It is not an operation to be undertaken lightly even now but now there is no doubt that it was performed successfully in prehistoric times.

Some skulls have been found on which the operation has been performed more than once. Doubtless many patients died, either from the operation itself or the disease that was being treated, but many certainly recovered. It is possible to tell by the growth of new bone around the edges of the hole that many of the patients recovered and lived for years afterwards. The illustration shows this very clearly. These skulls were found in a megalithic stone age grave in Denmark. Out of four hundred trephined skulls examined by one investigator, two hundred and fifty had certainly recovered from the operation.

Why the operation was done can only be guessed. Maybe it was performed then, as now, to relieve pressure on the brain, perhaps from a clot of blood following an injury; or in the hope of letting out demons or evil spirits. Whatever the reasons for the operation, it is surely interesting to know that even before men knew how to write they could operate on the human skull with only flint and later bronze and bone instruments.

To prove the effectiveness of these instruments, in 1962 Dr Grana of Peru operated on the skull of a thirty-one-year-old patient to remove a clot of blood which was causing paralysis following an injury to the head. The operation took place in a modern theatre with all the advantages of modern antiseptics and anaesthetics, but the surgeon's only instruments were prehistoric, illustrated opposite. The patient made a good recovery.

Much of what was believed was probably quite incorrect, but it is foolish to deduce from this that everything prehistoric man

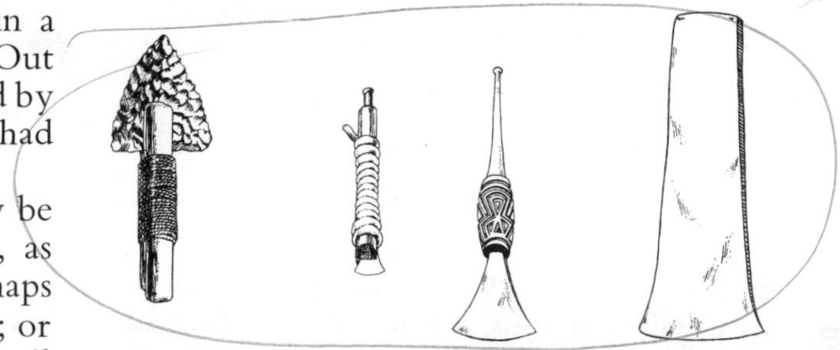

Stone and bronze instruments found in Peru

did was based on guesswork. Doubtless mistakes were made and wrong ideas believed then, as now, but, just as it is unwise to accept that because something has continued for a long time it cannot be improved, so also is it foolish to believe that only the new has value.

The history of medicine frequently shows that on the one hand skills and knowledge have not been developed because of an unwillingness to accept that established ideas might be wrong; and on the other that they have been lost because the new has been preferred to the old. This has not always been because the medical practitioners themselves have been retrogressive but because their actions have been limited by the ideas prevalent in the society in which they lived.

CHAPTER TWO
Early medicine in Egypt, India and China

In the fifth century BC, Herodotus, a Greek from Halicarnassus, wrote a book which has survived the passage of time. This book, although called *History of the Greek and Persian War*, is much more than the outline of a war. Herodotus travelled widely and the book contains a great deal of information about the way of life of people in the different countries that he visited. In a section describing Egypt and the Egyptians, he says:

> Medicine is practised among them on a plan of separation: each physician treats a single disorder, and no more: thus the country swarms with medical practitioners, some undertaking to cure diseases of the eye, others of the head, others again of the teeth, others of the intestines, and some those which are not local.

This suggests that medical practice in Egypt, at least as early as the fifth century BC, was already highly specialized.

About a hundred years later, Aristotle, who was the son of a physician and, amongst many things one of the earliest biologists, wrote:

> . . . Even in Egypt a doctor is allowed to depart from his textbook instructions if the patient is not well after four days . . .

This indicates a scientific practice of medicine based on recorded knowledge from the past. And so, after more than two thousand years, we are beginning to discover was the case, for, since the middle of the nineteenth century, more and more information has come to light regarding the practice of medicine in ancient times, especially in Egypt.

Very early in their civilization the Egyptians developed a method of writing. At first this was in a form known as hieroglyphics, which consisted of pictures representing words carved in stone as shown in the illustration on the next page. Soon, however,

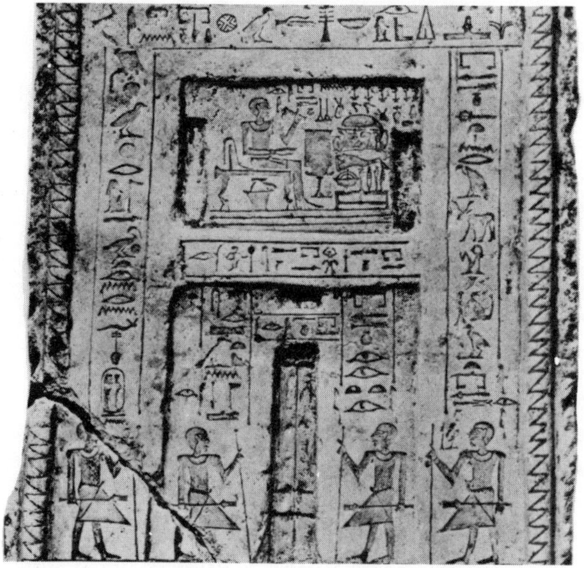

Stele of the Chief Court Physician, about 2600 BC

they discovered that the pith of papyrus reeds from the Nile, could be cut into strips and pressed between stones to make sheets of material like paper on which they could write. As it was much quicker to write on papyrus than carve words in stone they developed the hieratic script in which all the important medical papyri have been written.

The first of these papyri to be published in facsimile, although not the first to be discovered, was the *Ebers' Papyrus* in 1875 but it was not until 1890 that a first translation was made. Now nine important medical papyri are known, the oldest of which the *Kahoun Papyrus* dates from about 1950 BC. None of them is complete, although the *Ebers' Papyrus* is one hundred and eight pages long, and some are badly damaged. All of them are copies of older works and all still present some difficulties of translation.

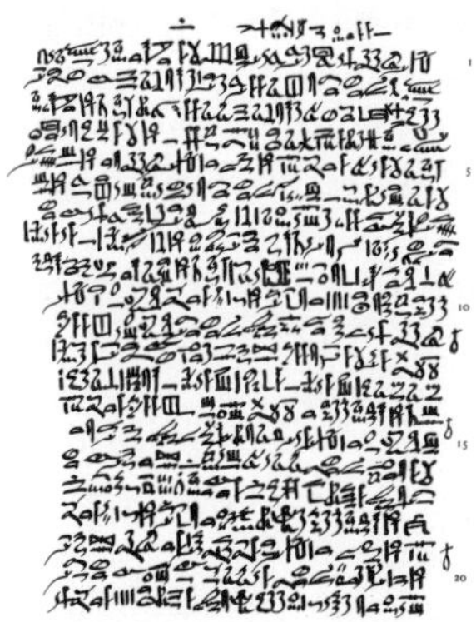

A section of the Ebers Papyrus written not later than 1555 BC

As well as these papyri Egyptologists (archaeologists and others concerned with the early history of Egypt) have discovered stone carvings, both of pictures and of writing, which give information dating from about 3000 BC. They provide us with evidence that in Egypt, more than two thousand years before Christ, a comprehensive system of medicine was practised which, although it contained a good deal of what we should today regard as magic, also shows evidence of intelligent observation and reasoning.

There were Houses of Life or pir-ankh which were medical centres of some sort. Perhaps they were hospitals, or medical schools or just surgeries; we do not know. But we do know that medical knowledge was available there and help was in some way provided from there when people were injured and ill. It seems quite likely that the House of Life was much more than merely a medical centre; it was probably rather more like a university today, where astronomy, mathematics and other sciences were studied as well as medicine. The *Kahoun Papyrus* for example, has a section on veterinary science and another on mathematics as well as a section on human medicine. It might perhaps have once been a book in the library of a House of Life.

It seems that physicians were often also priests: if not always at least frequently so.

> I am Chief of the Priests, Chief of the Magicians, Chief Physician to the King; who every day reads the books, who treats the sick, who lays his hand on the diseased whereby he knows them; gifted in the examination with the hand.

So said one called Heryshefnakht.

Imhotep has been called the first physician recognizable in history. He was Vizier to King Zozer in about 2800 BC and, as well as being a physician, he built one of the pyramids. He was later regarded by the Egyptians as a god and has been thought to be the origin of the Greek god Asklepios whom we shall encounter again in Chapter Three.

Whether the medical practitioner was priest or physician, or both, there is no doubt that some of the advice given and treatment recommended was good. The treatment recommended for a broken collar bone in an important surgical papyrus the *Edwin Smith Papyrus* is as good as could be given today. It was written perhaps five thousand years ago. Some people have even thought that it was written by Imhotep himself.

It was not only in Ancient Egypt that medicine had achieved standards that seem

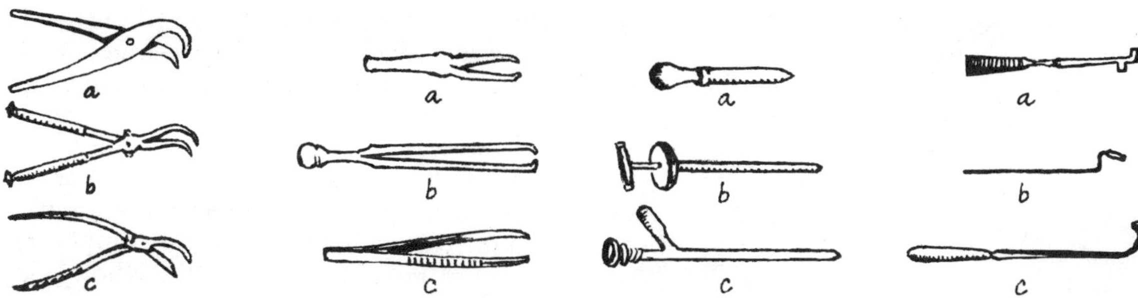

Comparison between Indian, Roman and modern instruments

surprising to the modern world. In India, hundreds of years before the birth of Christ, there were physicians and surgeons with skills that afterwards became lost to the world. Susruta, whose dates are uncertain but who practised in India certainly before 175 AD and probably much earlier, practised surgery which included at least operations for amputation of limbs, operations inside the abdomen, trephining the skull and operations on the nose. He described over one hundred surgical instruments and was aware of the need for cleanliness. Four instruments are illustrated (a) and compared with Roman (b) and modern (c) instruments for similar purposes. What anaesthetics were used we do not know, but some pain-deadening wines and powders were used.

At Tarila the present Rawalpindi there was a medical school. Hospitals were built by King Asoka more than two hundred years before the Christian era. In Ceylon it is recorded of a king, Duttha Gamani, that he

> daily maintained at eighteen different places, hospitals provided with suitable diet and medicines prepared by physicians for the infirm.

In China we also have some evidence of early medicine, but the predominating theory behind Chinese medicine has always been the balancing of the forces of Yin and Yang. It is not easy to explain what is meant by these forces but they have been regarded by the

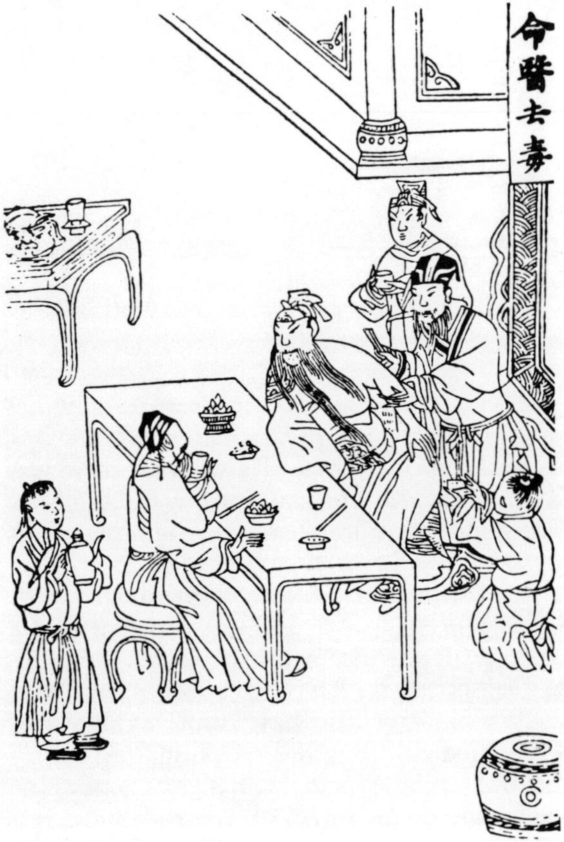

Hua To operating

Chinese as the essence of everything in the universe. When the forces become out of balance, disorder results. In the human being, when they are out of balance disease results and the way to restore health is to let out a little of the one which is in excess. For this purpose a system of medicine known as acupuncture developed. A most complicated system of lines of force over the whole body was developed and small needles were inserted beneath the skin. The diagnosis, as in all Chinese medicine, depended greatly on detailed observation of the pulse, and this decided the precise positioning of the needles and for how long they remained in place.

With one exception, however, there seems to have been almost no surgery in China until modern times. This might be because ancestor worship prevented anatomical dissection and thus prevented any real knowledge of anatomy. The one exception is a surgeon, Hua To, who is shown operating on an arrow wound in a Chinese general's arm. The general, having refused any pain-killing drugs, talks with a friend during the operation. This took place in the third century AD, and Hua To is the only recorded surgeon until approaching modern times.

CHAPTER THREE
Medicine in Ancient Greece and Rome

The most famous name in the history of medicine is that of a Greek, Hippocrates, who is known as the 'Father of Medicine'. He did not, however, invent medical practice.

Before Hippocrates' time medical practice in Greece centred in a religious cult, the cult of Asklepios, the Greek god of Medicine and the son of Apollo. Mythology tells us that Asklepios was saving so many lives that Pluto, the god of the Underworld, asked Zeus to slay him which Zeus did with a thunderbolt. Whatever the truth may be, whether Asklepios ever was a real man or not, by the fifth century BC there were many temples to Asklepios throughout the Greek world. Patients went to these temples where they spent the night and, whilst they slept, they perhaps dreamed. Sometimes Asklepios himself appeared to them in the dream. The priests at the temple would interpret the dreams and, by giving advice on the strength of their interpretation, guide the patients towards regaining their health.

One of the most famous Asklepions, the name given to temples dedicated to Asklepios, was at Epidaurus about fifty miles from Athens. This has been excavated and much interesting material found. The illustration on the next page is an artist's impression of the abaton at Epidaurus where the patients slept and achieved their cures. Many cases are recorded on stone tablets which have been found at Epidaurus. The case which is recounted below does not seem even to have needed the night's sleep:

> A dumb boy came as a suppliant to the temple to recover his voice. When he had performed the sacrifices and fulfilled the rites, the temple priest who bore the sacrificial fire turned to the boy's father and said, 'Do you promise to pay within a year the fee for the cure, if you obtain that for which you have come?' Suddenly the

boy answered 'I do.' His father was astonished at this, and told his son to speak again. The boy repeated the words and so was cured.

In an age when disease was looked upon as a punishment from the gods, it is not surprising that the best way of treating disease was thought to be that of offering sacrifices to the gods and appealing for their help.

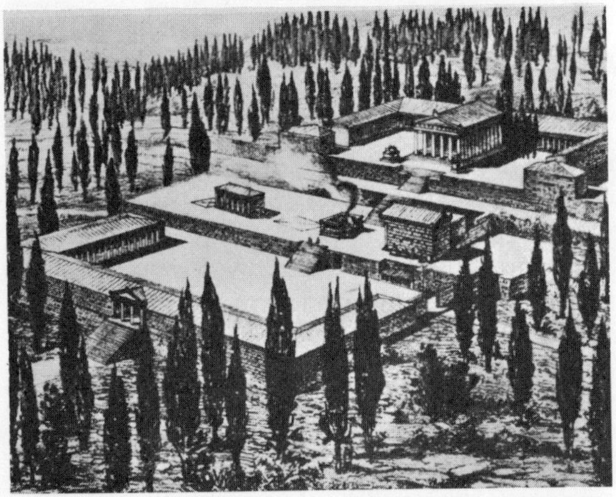

Artist's reconstruction of the Asklepion at Cos

Much of what we know of Asklepion medicine suggests magic rather than medicine but it must not be thought that this was necessarily so. Magic presupposes a magician, who achieves results by controlling supernatural powers, and there is no suggestion that this occurred. Miraculous cures are not quite the same thing. They are indeed the result of some powers which do not have obvious explanations. When they occur, as they do indeed occasionally today, it is often in people with great faith in their God. This is as likely to have been true two thousand five hundred years ago as it is today.

There are also people who suffer from a disease called hysteria in which some part of the body is unable to function although there is nothing wrong with the afflicted part itself. This is often due to emotional disturbances interfering with the nervous pathways and if the emotional blockage is overcome the part works again. Sudden cures are sometimes achieved in these illnesses and quite a lot of the recorded cures at Epidaurus might have been of this sort. The case mentioned of recovery from dumbness was probably one of these. The records of Epidaurus record only the successful cases and we cannot tell how many unsuccessful cases there were.

But quite apart from miracles or magic it is likely that many who visited the Asklepions would benefit from the common-sense advice given by the priests. Often the Asklepions were in the country and in healthy surroundings. Many patients probably benefited from the journey to them and possibly baths, exercises and massage, which were an important part of all cultured Greeks' lives, were available, and were all that was needed to make many of the patients well again.

It must not, however, be thought that this was the only medicine practised in Greece. There were also men who were more truly doctors, who devoted their lives to practising medicine and who developed a system of medicine which was based on reason. They practised the craft of medicine and were generally well regarded by the people.

In Greece craftsmen were not generally held in high esteem but they were respected for what they doubtless usually were, honest men doing a necessary job of work whether shoemaker, baker or physician. The physician was held perhaps in higher esteem because his craft or art was based on philosophy, or a knowledge of things and their causes, and demanded more than just technical skill.

These Greek physicians seemed to travel from place to place to find work, but certainly some Greek cities valued them highly enough to pay a salary to keep a particular physician in the city. Democedes was one of these and at different times he was state physician in Aegina, Athens and Samos. Many of these physicians, although not associated directly with Asklepions and certainly not Asklepion priests, were called Asklepiads. It seems likely that they looked upon Asklepios as their particular god, in the same ways as some people today look upon a patron saint. It was into this medical practice that Hippocrates came.

We do not know a great deal about the man himself except that he was born in Cos, a Greek island, in 460 BC and that he lived to be an old man, perhaps to the age of over a hundred. He travelled widely and the work that is in his name influenced the practice of medicine perhaps more than any other has ever done.

There are about seventy books attributed to Hippocrates and his followers. They are known as the *Hippocratic Collection* or *Corpus* and consist of textbooks on special subjects, lectures and notebooks. Although perhaps very few of these were actually the work of the Father of Medicine himself, they show the sort of approach that Hippocrates had to medicine and mark the beginnings of the medical practice known today. These books emphasize that disease is a natural phenomenon and not a punishment from a petulant god, that the natural course of disease should be observed, and that nature is a great healer and should not be interfered with if all is going well. They lay down many sound principles of medical practice and state what the ideals of a practitioner should be. The Hippocratic Oath, perhaps the best known of all the Hippocratic writings, states what is generally believed to be the ideal on which all medical practitioners should base their conduct. Although this is not now taken by doctors in many places, its principles still apply.

> I swear by Apollo the physician, by Asklepios . . . and by all the gods and goddesses . . . to hold my teacher in this art equal to my own parents . . . to impart precept, oral instruction, and all other instruction to my own sons, the sons of my teacher, and to indentured pupils who have taken the physician's oath, but to nobody else. I will use treatment to help the sick according to my ability and judgement, but never with a view to injury and wrong-doing. Neither will I administer a poison to anybody when asked to do so, nor will I suggest such a course. . . . I will keep pure and holy both my life and my art. . . . Into whatsoever houses I enter, I will enter to help the sick, and I will abstain from all intentional wrong-doing and harm . . . whatsoever I shall see or hear in the course of my profession, as well as outside my profession in my intercourse with men, if it be what should not be published abroad, I will never divulge, holding such things to be holy secrets. Now if I carry out this oath, and break it not, may I gain for ever reputation among all men for my life and for my art; but if I transgress it and forswear myself, may the opposite befall me.

The generally accepted explanation of man and his nature was that everything consisted of the elements fire, air, water and earth, and that in man these corresponded to the four humours of yellow bile, blood, phlegm, and black bile which in turn had the qualities of hot, cold, dry and wet in varying relationships with one another. Aristotle, born in 384 BC when Hippocrates was an old man, indicated the relationship by the diagram on page 17.

So long as these elements, humours and qualities were in the right proportions, good health resulted but, if they became unbalanced due to an excess or shortage of one or more of the humours, then disease resulted. It was

Ambroïse Paré performing an operation during the siege of Metz in 15

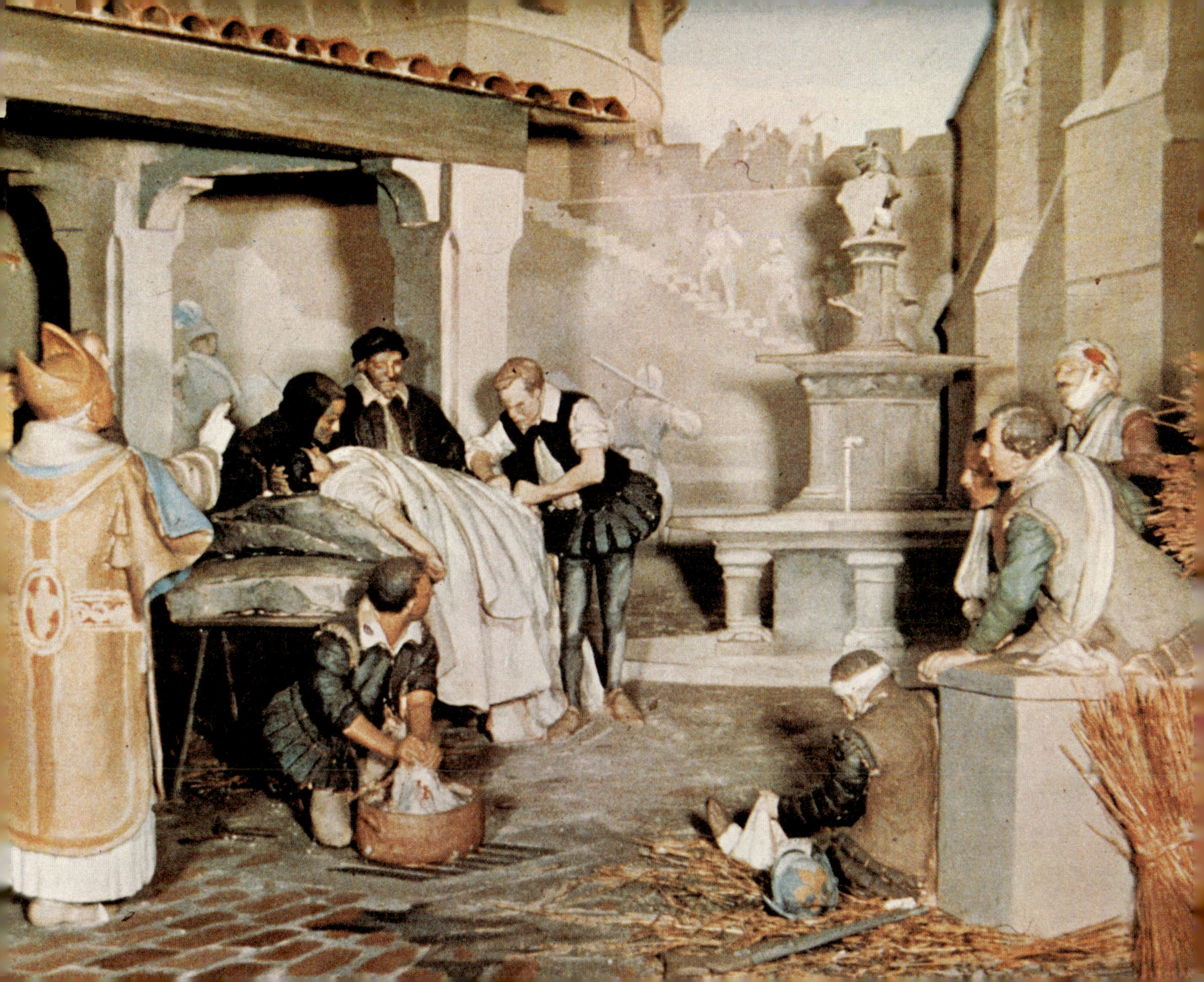

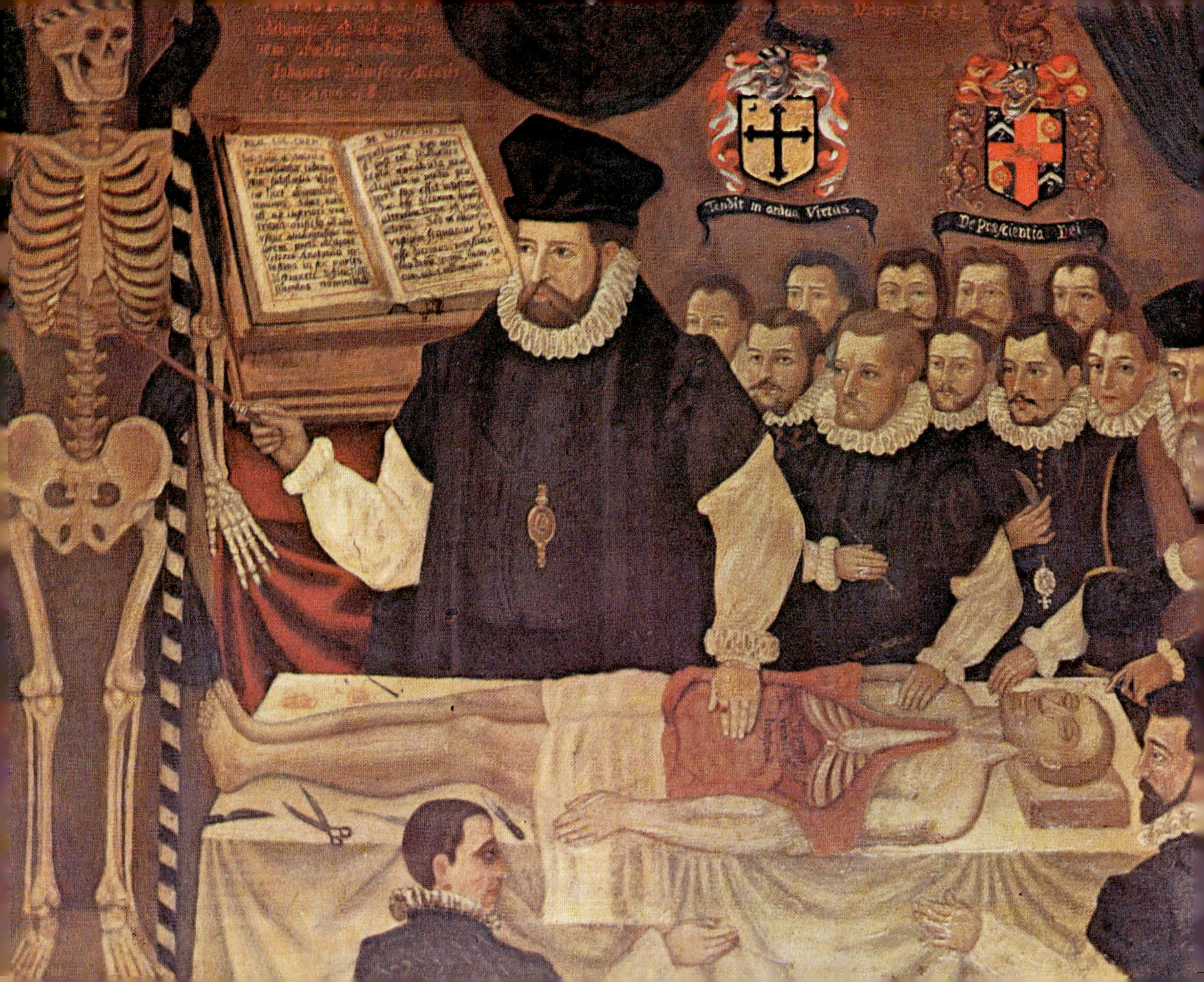
Tendit in ardua Virtus.
De Præscientia Dei

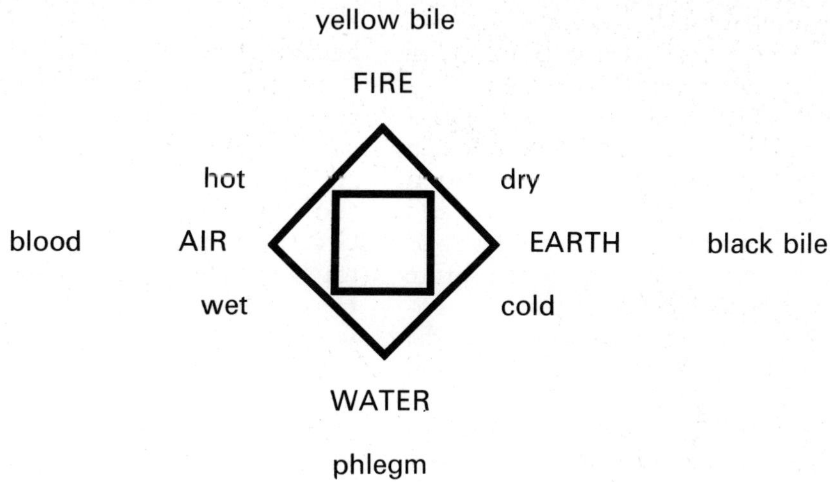

the physician's task to decide where the fault lay and to attempt to restore the balance. It is interesting here to recall the Chinese ideas about the forces of Yin and Yang and how disease resulted if they became out of balance which was mentioned in Chapter Two.

Hippocrates accepted the principle of the humours but he believed that given time nature tended to correct the imbalance when it occurred and that he should help nature only if necessary. To this end Hippocrates believed strongly that it was necessary for physicians to observe the natural course of disease and so be able to give a prognosis, that is foretell how the disease would progress. Only if the prognosis was unfavourable should the physician intervene and then only to help nature and not to usurp the natural healing processes.

Hippocrates became the Father of Medicine not so much because of what he did but because of his attitude towards medicine. He regarded his profession as a means of helping those in need by observation and rational action rather than by means of magic, as a

ıe new anatomy being taught at the Barber Surgeon's Hall in London, 1581.

means of helping the sick and not of glorifying himself, as a way of service to humanity and not domination over them.

He lived at a time when the Greek world was becoming the centre of civilization, when men were breaking away from superstition and magic and substituting observation and reason, when great thinkers such as Plato and Aristotle were emerging and when brute force was giving place to intelligent co-operation between men. Eventually the Roman Empire was to submerge Greece and was itself to be submerged by its own weaknesses. This, however, lay centuries ahead and in the third and second centuries BC Greek physicians were held in esteem and Greek medicine was honoured.

During the second century BC Alexandria in Egypt became the centre of Greek learning as a result of a school of medicine being founded there in 300 BC under Ptolemy, the ruler, and for hundreds of years a medical education at Alexandria was perhaps a guarantee of medical employment throughout the Roman Empire. This is how it came about.

Egypt had been conquered by Alexander the Great and on his death it came under the rule of the Greek Ptolemy who was one of Alexander the Great's generals. Alexandria became a favourite residence of this Greek dynasty and under it the town became more Greek than Egyptian. Ptolemy and his successors were patrons of learning and at the Alexandrian School remarkable anatomical and physiological researches were made by Greek physicians. The two earliest medical teachers at Alexandria were also the greatest, Herophilus of Chalcedon and the slightly younger Erasistratus of Chios.

Herophilus may be regarded as the founder of anatomy, Erasistratus as the founder of physiology. They carried out post-mortem examinations on human beings perhaps for the first time. It is also said that they practised vivisection but this is not necessarily true. It should be remembered that, terrible as it may sound today, torture was a part of life and to both doctors and criminals it might have seemed a kindness to permit experimental operations under the effects of pain-relieving drugs rather than submit to other horrifying tortures. The anatomy and physiology propounded by these men was far from the truth as we know it today, but it was an attempt to base understanding on firsthand experience and reality.

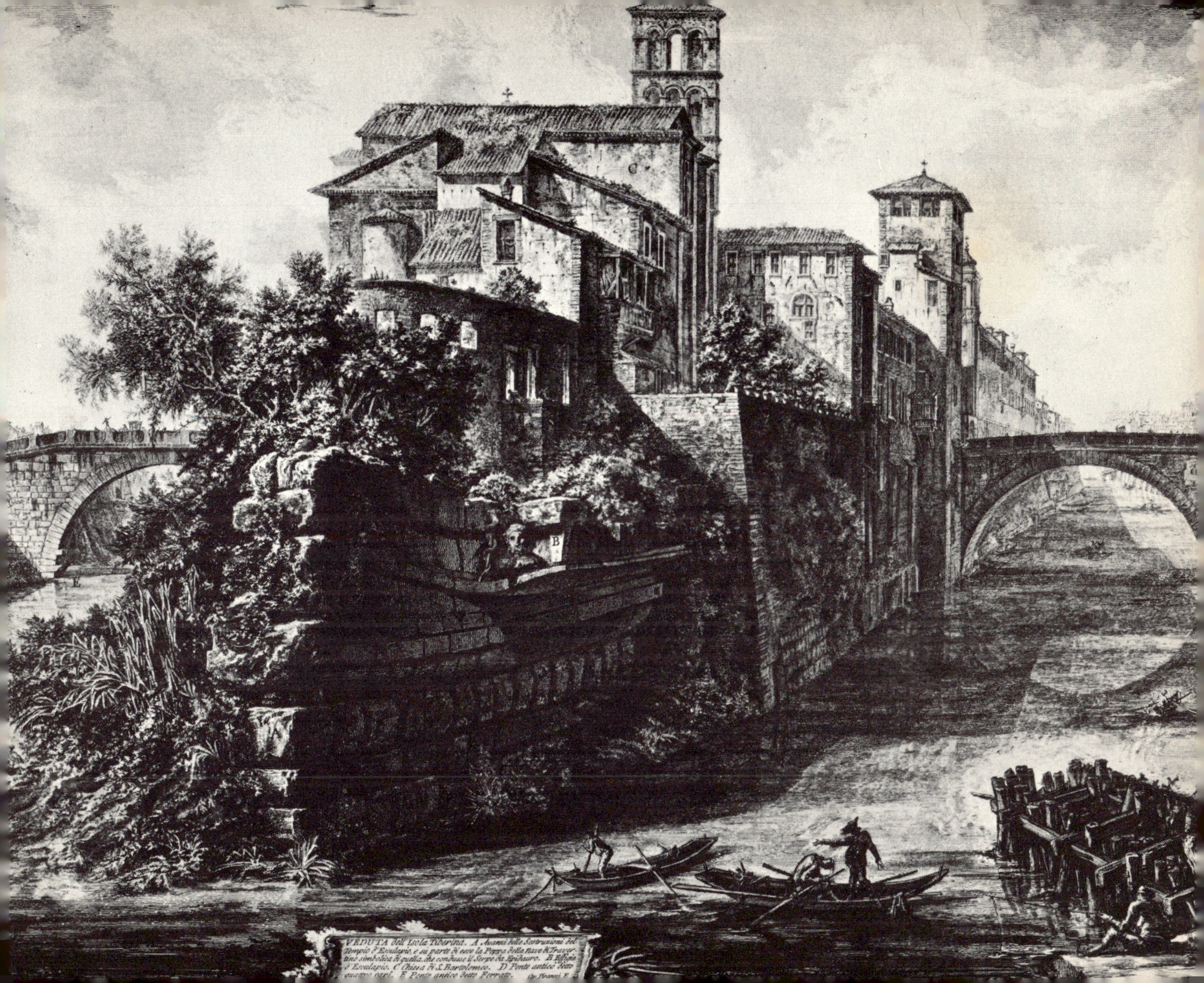
VEDUTA dell'Isola Tiberina. A Avanzi delle Sostruzioni del
Tempio d'Esculapio, e su parte di esse la Poppa della Nave di Traver-
tino simbolica di quella, che condusse il Serpe da Epidauro. B Effigie
d'Esculapio. C Chiesa di S. Bartolomeo. D Ponte antico detto
quattro capi. E Ponte antico detto Ferrato.
Piranesi F.

Through the school at Alexandria much medical practice found its way to Rome.

Although the Roman Empire, which, with all its shortcomings, was one of the great civilizing influences in Europe and throughout the world, produced two of the famous or infamous names in medical history, it contributed little in the way of new thought to the practice of medicine between doctor and patient. What did come from Rome was the beginnings of organization and administration of medical services and especially the establishment of hospitals.

Sanitation and some control of public health matters were the concern of the Romans from very early times. Some of the great sewers of Rome, built several hundred years BC, still exist and at least until recently were in use. Fresh water was brought to Rome via the aqueducts at the rate of hundreds of millions of gallons per day. Laws were enacted as early as 450 BC regulating burials. By AD 160 public physicians were appointed whose duties included provision of medical aid to the poor.

One hospital, or valetudinarium as the Romans called it, was established on an island in the Tiber probably as early as 290 BC. Legend has it that the Romans sent a party of men to Delphi for advice from the oracle regarding the health of the people of Rome. The party brought back a sacred snake (for sacred snakes were always associated with the Asklepiadiae) which escaped from the boat as it was approaching Rome up the Tiber. The snake swam ashore to the island which thus became a recognized place to seek for health. The illustration on page 19, which is by Piranesi, shows how the island appeared in the eighteenth century.

It was on this island that a church to St Bartholomew was built and, in the twelfth century AD, a monk from there called Rahere came to England and founded St Bartholomew's Hospital in London. Thus its origin can be traced to the oracle at Delphi. Also, infirmaries were established for the sick slaves to go to, perhaps to end their days without being a direct burden to their owners but at least without being cast out to die on the streets of Rome.

In addition to the hospitals established for the civil population, the Romans also made provisions for the care of their soldiers. A military hospital near Dusseldorf about AD 100 has been excavated.

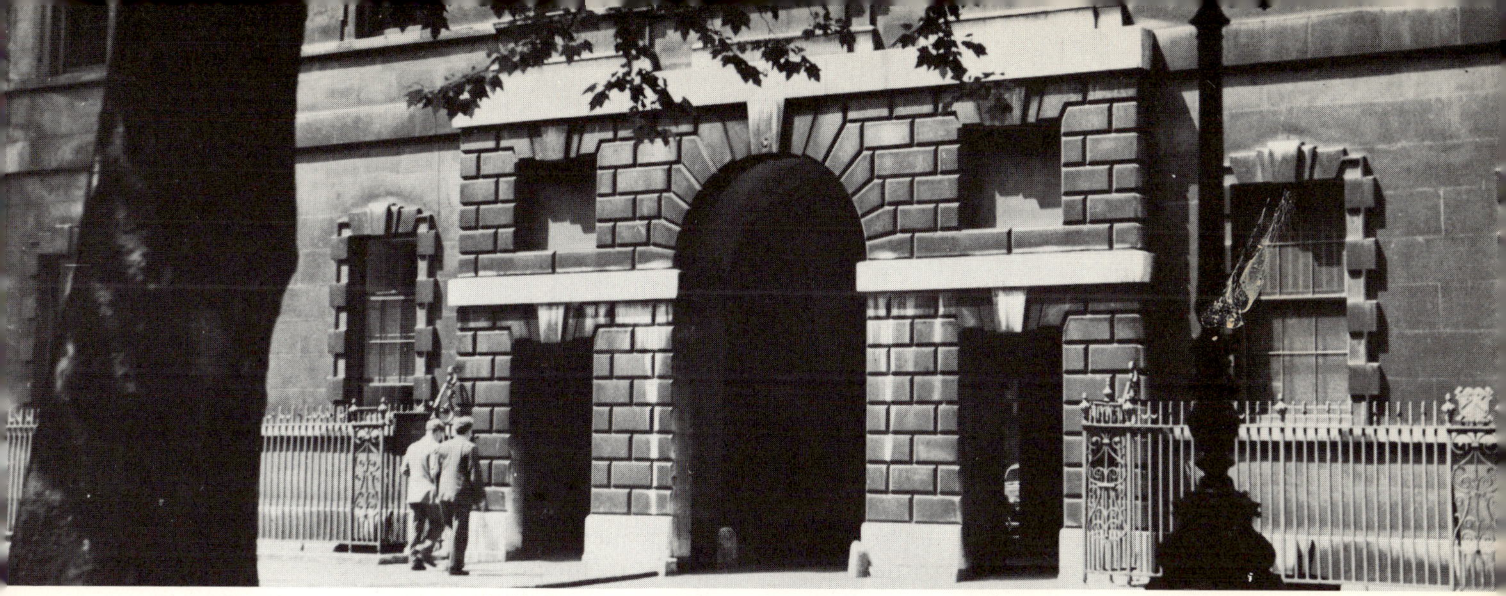

The front of St Bartholomew's Hospital as it is today

Two names stand out from Roman medical history, Galen and Celsus. Celsus, born about AD 10, composed a sort of general encyclopaedia. The only part which has survived is that concerned with medicine and it tells us what medical knowledge was known at the time. Celsus was not himself a physician.

The other was Galen whose name is still preserved in certain types of medicines known as galenicals today. Galen, AD 129–199, was not a Roman but he came to Rome after visiting many medical centres. He wrote a great deal and his ideas, although often quite wrong, became the accepted teaching throughout the medical schools of Europe for over a thousand years. He was famous in Rome during his lifetime and was undoubtedly both learned and clever. He seems, nevertheless, to have been far from modest and frequently recounts examples of his own cleverness. His descriptions of the anatomy of the human body lasted until Vesalius, whom we shall meet in Chapter Five, proved him wrong in the sixteenth century.

CHAPTER FOUR
Mainly Arabic medicine

From the fall of the Roman Empire in Europe in the fifth century until the Renaissance, which for medicine began in the sixteenth century, no progress was made in Europe either in medical knowledge or in its practice. Instead of the ordered way of life brought by the Romans there was the disorder of barbarism. The general conditions of life in Europe were not those in which learning could flourish, nor even readily survive. But what centralized order there was lay in the unity of the Christian church.

From the beginning of the sixth century the monasteries began to develop. In AD 529 Benedict founded the monastery of Monte Casino and, although this was not the earliest monastery in Europe, it was the beginnings of the type that was to spread throughout Europe in the succeeding centuries.

Although the original purpose of the monastic life was that of prayer and not of scholarship, the monasteries gradually became the centres of scholarship and learning. It was practically only in these centres that reading and writing could be learned or practised. Their scholarship, however, was not particularly or even very much concerned with medicine. The studies, other than theology and biblical studies, mentioned in the records of one early important monastery were grammar, rhetoric, dialectic, arithmetic, geometry, astronomy and music, there is no mention of medicine.

Nonetheless, it was in these centres that some medical manuscripts were preserved and copied and, because they were the only centres of learning, it was only through the monasteries that the little medical knowledge that did survive in Europe survived at all.

The monks, however, did nothing to advance medicine. In places they practised it because there was no one else to do so, but progress was halted, and because there was no real interest, in many ways it degenerated and regressed. There was no intellectual curiosity, no spirit of enquiry, only a rule of thumb application of what fragments were remembered from the past.

During this time the real history of medicine is almost wholly to be found in the medical practice of the Arabs. It is so called because almost all the new writing of this time was in Arabic and the majority of the practitioners were Muslims. Some of these writings were translations of Greek and Roman authors and did not originate from the Arabian schools. It is, however, because they were translated and used that they survived for future generations. There they were studied and used in practice, by men who were doctors and not monks, in a way that was never the case in the monasteries of Europe. The Arabs kept alive what had developed in the ancient world whilst Europe generally lapsed into barbarism.

European learning reached into Persia as the result of persecution in the Christian church. A large section of the early Christian church, called Nestorians after their leading bishop, Nestorius, fled to Persia and with them went both manuscripts and the ability to translate them into the language of their new country. They were welcomed into Persia perhaps because both had the common enemy of Rome. Persia was afraid of the Eastern Roman Empire and the Nestorians of the Roman Christianity.

In the early part of the seventh century a further event occurred which at first had no relationship with medical practice at all. This was the rise of Islam. It began with the prophet Mohammed, and the Muslim religion is considered as dating from AD 622. The religious movement spread rapidly and in the next 110 years the Arabs set forth to conquer most of North Africa along the Mediterranean shore. At the Straits of Gibraltar they crossed to Spain and advanced into France where they were at last halted in 732 by Charles Martel at Tours. They retreated behind the Pyrenees but Spain, North Africa and much of what is now the Middle East remained as the Muslim Empire.

After this first zeal the Arabs turned some of their energy to less warlike pursuits and the study and practice of medicine spread throughout the Muslim world – from Mesopotamia in the east to Spain in the west.

The progress of medicine in this time was due at least as much to the wisdom of the ruling Caliphs and Sultans as to the physicians themselves. In the east, at Baghdad, the Caliphs encouraged libraries and supported hospitals. Jundisapur - which no longer exists but which was once near to Baghdad - was the centre of medical learning.

At Cordova in Spain, which was the capital of the Western Caliphate, there are said to have been fifty well-run hospitals. Although this may be an over-estimate, certainly hospitals, together with schools and libraries, were encouraged and supported by the rulers.

Much Arabian medicine, whether practised by Persian, Egyptian, Jew or Spaniard, developed from the learning that had been acquired by translation of Greek and perhaps Hindu manuscripts at Jundisapur.

Since dissection of human bodies after death was not approved by the Muslim faith, knowledge of anatomy was still inaccurate and physiology the guesswork of the past.

These Arabian physicians, however, were observant and it was Abdallatif, when in Egypt, who first questioned the accuracy of Galen. He discovered a vast graveyard of skeletons and observed that, although Galen had said that there were two bones in the lower jaw, all the skeletons had lower jaws consisting of one bone only.

It was the Arabian physicians also who originated the apothecaries, and the first pharmacopoea, which is a book listing medicines with instructions for their use, came from Jundisapur.

In the west, Rhazes and Avicenna - whose full names are much longer and more complicated - wrote works which survived and were used for centuries. Rhazes gave the first recorded descriptions of smallpox and measles in the Western world and introduced many remedies into medicine, particularly mercurial ointments.

In Egypt, Isaac ben Solomon, a Jew, wrote *The Physician's Guide*. One quotation from this, 'When a patient can be cured by diet use no drug, and when simple medicines suffice avoid complicated ones' is just as good advice to-day as it was a thousand years ago, and is indeed the teaching of Hippocrates.

In the west, Albucassis (also spelt Abulcassis), who probably died at the age of one hundred and one in the year 1013, wrote the first illustrated book on surgery. He knew and said that there was much ignorance of

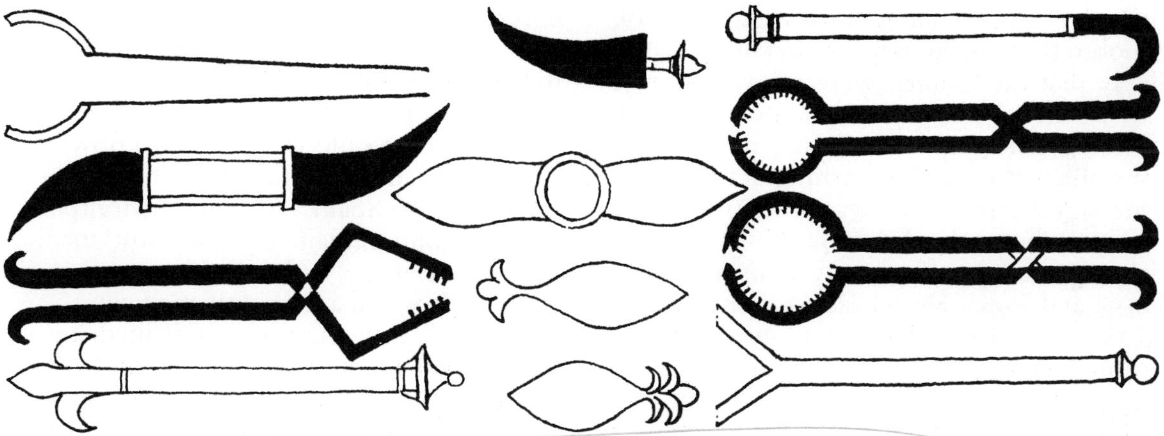

A drawing of some instruments shown in Albucassis's book

anatomy but, nevertheless, his book was used extensively by surgeons for very many years. The picture shows a selection of instruments as illustrated in this work.

The fund of knowledge, held in store by the Arabian physicians from Greece, Rome and perhaps a little from India, and added to by their own observations, was the basis from which European medicine of the early Middle Ages grew.

In Europe itself, however, there was one place where a medical school did arise in the ninth or tenth century. This was at Salerno in Southern Italy. Not very much is known about this school but, although it had connections with the monastery of Montecassino, there were doctors who were not also priests or monks. It is also possible that there were women doctors. Certainly there were 'the ladies of Salerno', one of whom named Trotula is said to have written a book on obstetrics. Although not certain, it seems likely that the women were midwives only.

This school, although not directly Arabian at all, did act as a portal of entry into Europe for some of the medical learning of the Arabs. One significant figure was Constantine the African who, in the eleventh century, came to Salerno after spending many years in Africa, Persia and India. He translated many Arabic works into Latin including some of the original Greek medical manuscripts which might otherwise have been lost to Europe.

This medical school at Salerno continued to flourish for several centuries and it was the world centre of medical learning in about AD 1200. After this, however, it rapidly declined although it continued to exist until closed formally by decree of Napoleon in 1811. It is said that at Salerno the description or title of doctor first came into use. There is now no trace of where the medical school existed.

As the importance of Salerno declined, so did other centres arise. Montpellier in south-eastern France became, for a time, the foremost centre in the world. This was perhaps because it is almost a meeting-place between northern Italy and Spain. Then new ideas were just beginning to develop in the northern Italian centres of learning. Montpellier was a health resort and would doubtless have patients who would seek both the knowledge from Italy and the practice of the Arabs as preserved in Spain. Although Montpellier did not long remain the foremost medical centre of Europe, it did not disappear as did Salerno. It is still a school of medicine.

The early influences of Arabic medicine on Britain and the rest of Europe, and of the new thought from Italy, was via Montpellier.

There were medical practitioners in Britain but none of great significance. It was not to be until the sixteenth and seventeenth centuries that Britain was to begin to come to the fore in the history of the progress of medicine.

In the thousand years between AD 500 and AD 1500 medical practice gained little. There were, so far as we know, and it is unlikely that all traces would have been lost, no real centres of medical learning other than Salerno and, later, Montpellier. Towards the end of this time, however, fresh interest was beginning to arise and ever since then progress has been more and more rapid.

CHAPTER FIVE
Vesalius, Harvey and the beginnings of scientific medicine

Anatomy is the science of the structure of the body and physiology the science of how it works. Although it is convenient to consider them as separate sciences, they are each essential to the proper understanding of the human being both in health and in disease. Unless one knows what is normal one cannot tell what is abnormal and unless one knows how a thing is constructed one cannot know how it works.

For many reasons, some of which have been mentioned already, there were major obstacles to dissection of the human body in the Middle Ages and earlier. These obstacles did not suddenly disappear in the fifteenth and sixteenth centuries; there was still much prejudice against dissection and there was difficulty in obtaining suitable bodies, but men were becoming less inclined to accept what ancient writers had said and more inclined to look for themselves.

The teaching of anatomy up to this time had been based on the writings of Galen, writings dating from the second century. He wrote in Greek, but later his writings were translated into Arabic and, often via Arabic, into Latin. Every copy was done laboriously by hand. Every time a copy was made mistakes were also likely to be made – and, of course, the mistake copied on the next occasion with further mistakes creeping in. After more than a thousand years it could hardly be expected that what Galen had written originally was still presented accurately. When it is further realized that much of Galen's anatomy was based on the pig (thought to be similar to the human being) it is not surprising that much was wrong.

The accepted method of teaching medicine was for the professor to read from Galen and an assistant to cut the body to demonstrate what was there, which did not encourage students to discover for themselves. So it was until Vesalius came on the scene.

Andreas Vesalius, born in Brussels in 1514, studied at Louvain and then at Paris. In Paris he managed to secure the job of actually dissecting a body whilst the professor read from Galen. What he saw for himself convinced him that further investigation was necessary. He went to Padua in Italy and in 1538, at the youthful age of twenty-four, was appointed professor of anatomy.

During the next five years he worked diligently to discover for himself as much of the truth about the human body as he could and, in 1543, he published these findings in a book *De humani corporis fabrica (The Fabric of the Human Body)*. This book is perhaps the most important single work affecting the progress of medicine that has ever been published. What Vesalius discovered was important, but of even greater importance was that he proved by his own research that the ancient authorities, particularly Galen, were wrong about many things. What for centuries had been assumed to be true because the ancient authorities said it was so was now shown by Vesalius to be inaccurate.

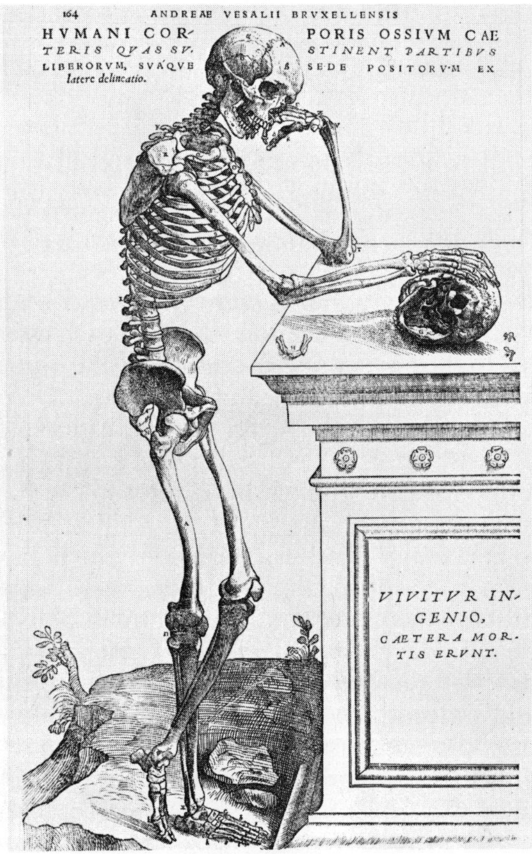

From 'De humani corporis fabrica'

... For I am not unaware of how much disturbance the doctors ... raise when they observe that Galen deviated more than two hundred times from the correct description of the harmony, use, and function of the parts of man in treatment of anatomy alone, as I now exhibit it in the schools, while they examine sharply the dissected particles with the greatest zeal in defending him. Although these men, led by the love of truth, gradually grow milder and put a little more trust in their rational faculties and their eyes – by no means ineffectual eyes and brains – than to the writings of Galen, ...

If Galen could be wrong in some places, men began to argue, he could be wrong in others. If Galen could be wrong, then so could other ancient authorities. If this was so then there was good reason for finding out for oneself, not accepting something because it had been believed for a thousand years, but only if it could be shown to be true.

Although it is not strictly history of medicine, perhaps we should note that also in 1543 Copernicus showed that the earth moved round the sun and not the sun round the earth.

Vesalius' work (and Copernicus' as well) was to influence men more quickly because of the relatively new invention, printing.

Printing was invented in Germany about 1440. It was therefore still in its infancy, but nevertheless it was possible to produce several copies of a manuscript quicker and more accurately than by hand. This is especially important when, as with Vesalius' book, so much of the information is conveyed by drawings, and Vesalius was perhaps lucky to have such fine engraving on the anatomical plates. The book was printed by Joannes Oporinus in Basle in Switzerland where Vesalius himself went to superintend the work. The illustration of the complete human skeleton taken from Vesalius' book gives some idea of the thoroughness and accurate attention to detail which prevails throughout the book. This is especially noticeable when one compares this illustration with the fourteenth century drawing on the next page of a skeleton from a manuscript in a French museum.

Another man, much better known today, had dissected and drawn human anatomy some thirty years earlier than Vesalius.

This gentleman has compiled a particular treatise of anatomy, with the demonstration in draft not only of the members, but also of the

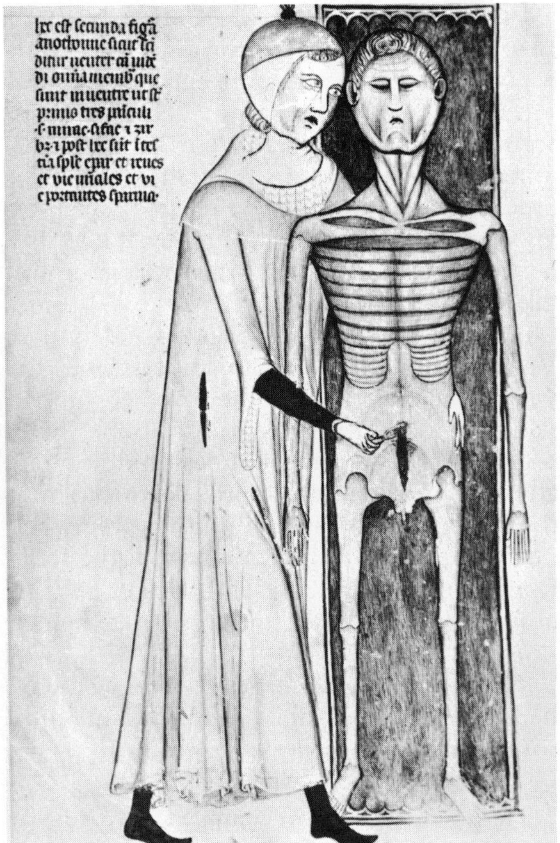

Fourteenth century drawing of the skeleton

> muscles, nerves, joints, intestines, and of whatever can be reasoned about in the bodies both of men and women, in a way that has never yet been done by any other person. All of which we have seen with our own eyes; and he said that he has already dissected more than thirty bodies, both men and women of all ages.

These words were written by Antonio de Beatis about Leonardo da Vinci after he had paid da Vinci a visit on 10th October 1517. But da Vinci's anatomical drawings were stored away for two hundred years before being re-discovered. Many of them are now in the Royal Collection at Windsor Castle.

However brilliant Leonardo's work in anatomy it was unknown until long after Vesalius had published his work on anatomy. Although perhaps one of the most gifted men who has ever lived, Leonardo da Vinci has not directly influenced the course of medicine at all. What his place might have been in the history of medicine if his work had been published we do not know.

Although anatomy is the science of the structure of the body, and physiology the science of how it works, Vesalius and his contemporaries were not satisfied with understanding the structure. They were also concerned with how things worked. Despite this, it was to be another eighty-five years before the first major breakthrough in physiology occurred and the information published.

We speak to-day of the circulation of the blood as though it is a self-evident fact; as though it is obvious that the blood goes round the body in a continuous motion. It is, indeed, now almost self-evident but only because of the knowledge we have gained from the past. Even in Ancient Egypt it was known that the pulse indicated something of the state of the heart as this extract shows.

> When any physician . . . applies . . . his fingers (to the various pulses) . . . then he examines the heart, because all his limbs possess its vessels, that is, it speaks out of the vessels of every limb . . .

But the fact that the blood circulated was not known for more than another three and a half thousand years. Before that it was thought that the blood, mixed with certain vital spirits, was pumped with a sort of to-and-fro motion along the arteries. This is not so surprising when one realizes that to the naked eye there is no connection at all between arteries and veins for the capillaries are too small to be seen without a microscope.

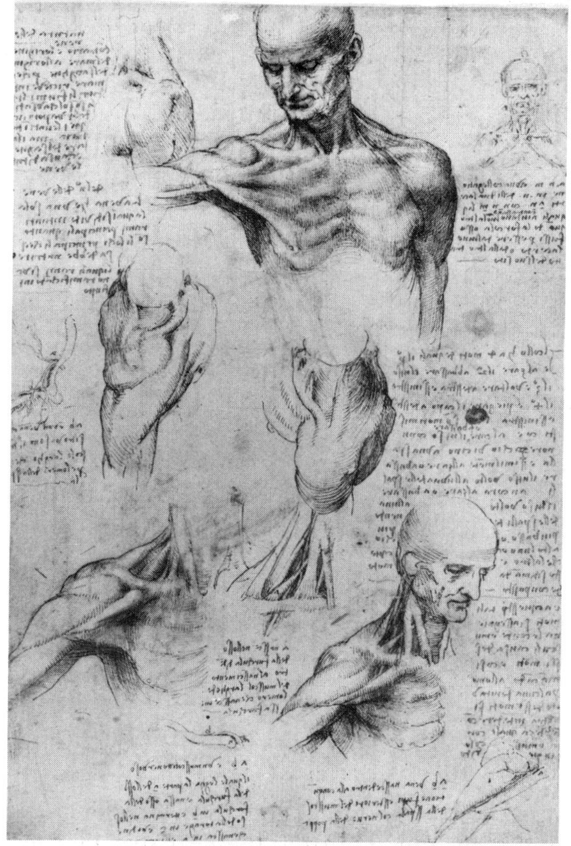

Some of da Vinci's anatomical drawings

It was not until the work of William Harvey, an Englishman born in Folkestone, that the circulation of the blood was scientifically shown to be a fact, proved by experiment, and established as the basis of physiology. In 1628 Harvey published *An Anatomical Disquisition on the Movement of the Heart and Blood in Animals*. In this, for the first time, it was argued that, from the observed facts, the same blood must be pumped through the heart time and time again. By calculating the weight of blood expelled by the heart in half an hour, he showed that only if the same blood was used over and over again could the amount needed possibly be made available; and he demonstrated by simple experiments how the blood flowed out from the heart along the arteries and back again via the veins.

How the blood passed from the arteries to the veins Harvey did not know. To discover the capillaries he needed the microscope which had yet to be invented. Without it he assumed that the blood must diffuse through the tissues and be collected up by the veins.

The discovery of the capillaries was made thirty or more years later by Marcello Malpighi, an Italian born in the year that Harvey published his book, 1628, and independently by a Dutchman, Antonj van Leeuwenhoek, who made many of the early discoveries in all sorts of fields using the microscope.

> I have said before that the corpuscles or globules that make the blood red, are so small that ten hundred thousand of them are not so big as a grain of coarse sand, and so we easily imagine how very small the blood-vessels are in which the circulation of the blood takes place. . . . These blood-vessels (that is, the capillaries) were exceedingly numerous. . . . All these vessels were so small or thin that no more than one corpuscle could pass through it at a time . . .

Thus began scientific anatomy and physiology upon which the whole of modern medicine and surgery has been built.

Vesalius showed that the way to knowledge was to observe for oneself. Harvey showed how observation and measurement could lead one to deductions which could be tested and proved by experiment. Malpighi and van Leeuwenhoek extended the ability to see smaller structures than was possible with the unaided senses by using the (then modern) microscope and, in so doing, they opened up greater fields of study for anatomists and provided the missing evidence to prove the accuracy of Harvey's work.

An operation as it appeared in Lister's day; note the carbolic spr

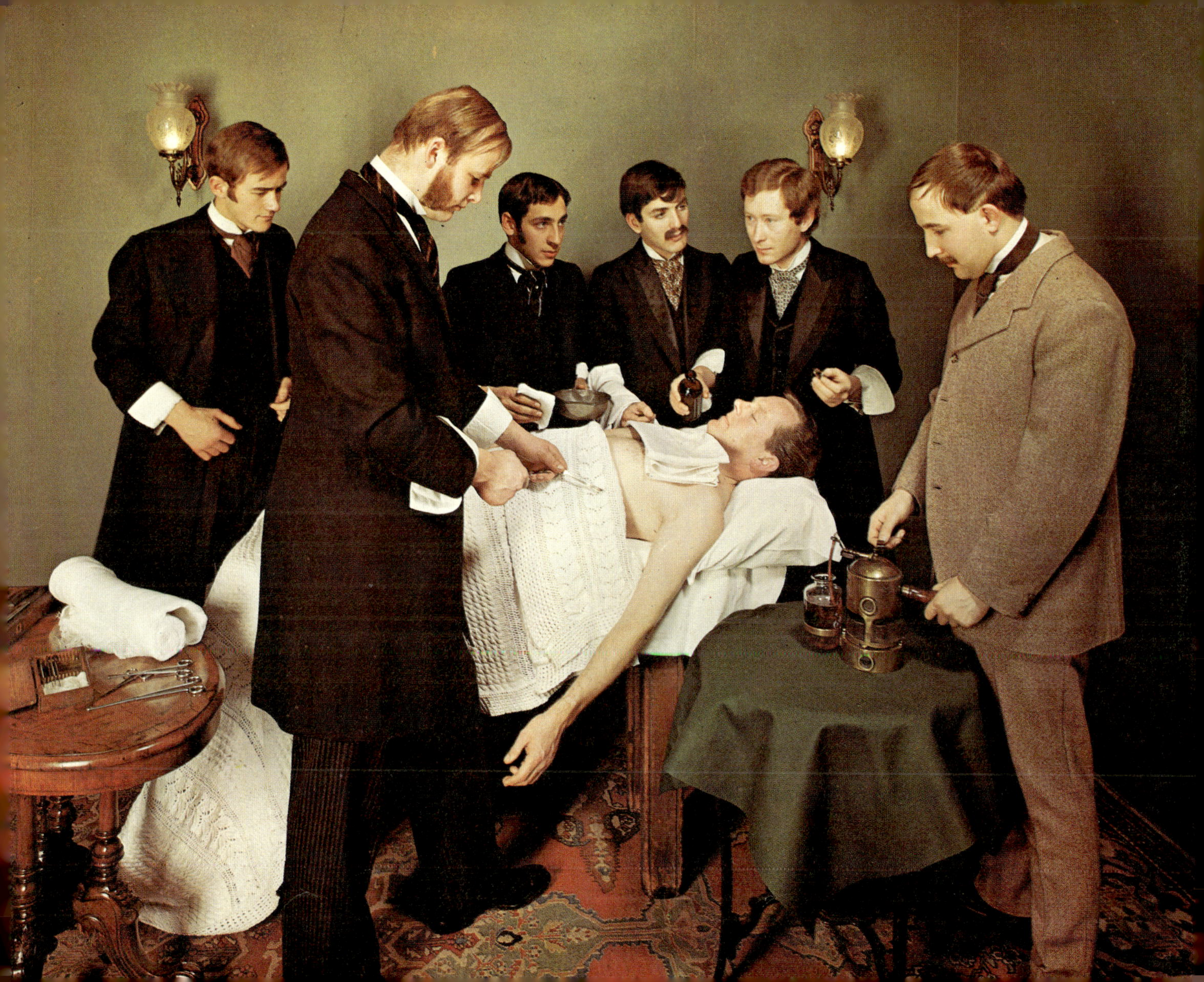

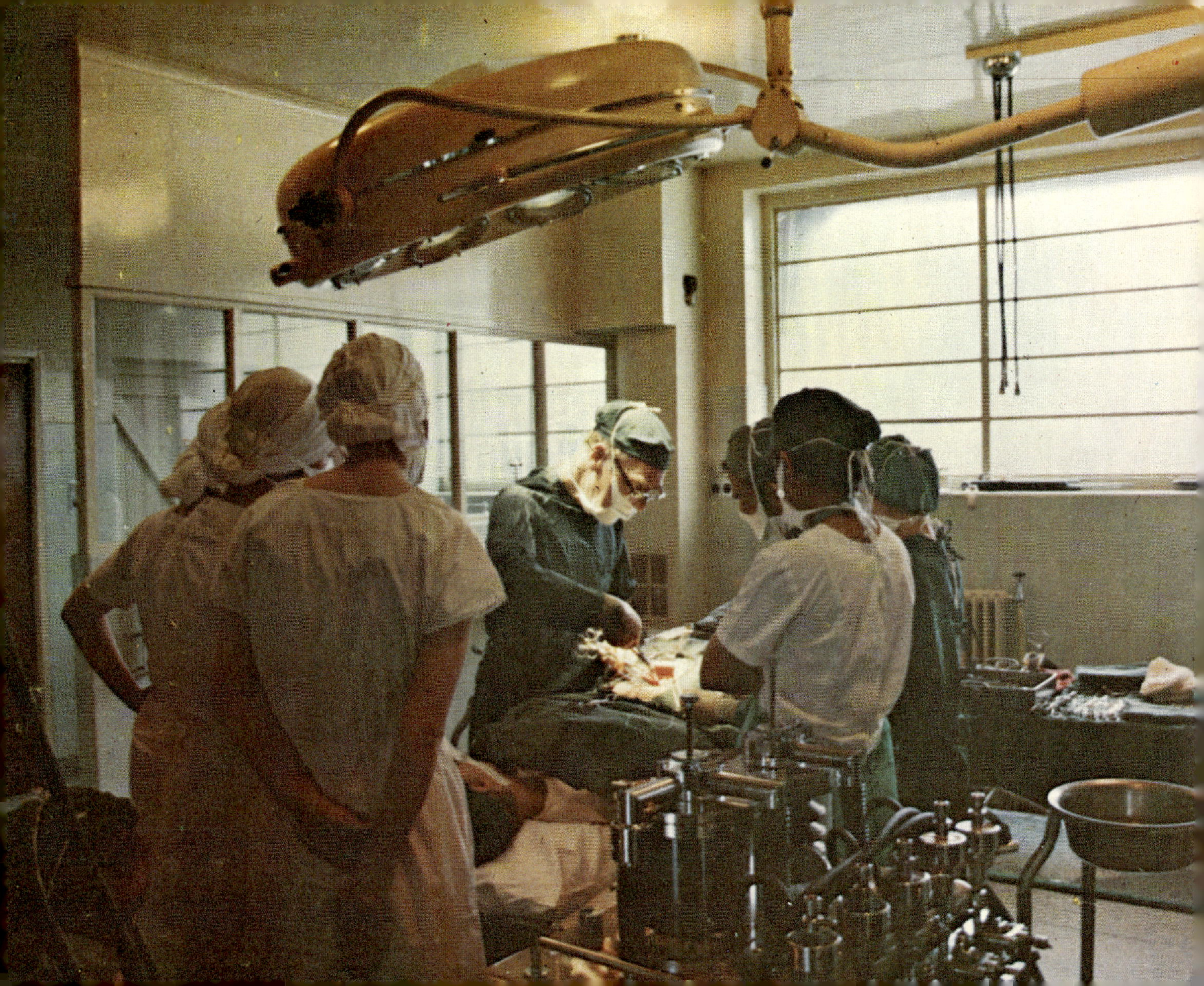

CHAPTER SIX
Mechanical aids in medicine

In every human being there is a body, a mind and a spirit or soul. Of these parts it may be that the spirit or soul is the most important, the body and the mind being but temporary coverings for the soul to inhabit whilst on earth but, whether this is so or not, it is the body and the mind with which medicine is now principally concerned. As we have seen, this has not always been the case and, although there are many people today who believe still that body, mind and soul cannot be regarded separately, the spiritual side of man is generally regarded as being outside medical practice and in the domain of the priest.

Now whatever else the human being might be, he is at least a very complicated piece of machinery, and a piece of working machinery. It is when something goes wrong with the machine of the body or mind that a human being is regarded as ill and in need of medical help to return to health. It is the business of the doctor to discover what it is that has gone wrong and to provide what help he can to put things right. The doctor makes a diagnosis and advises treatment.

Although every human being is different from every other in some respects, yet in others they are similar. For example, although no one has the same fingerprints as anyone else, almost everyone has four fingers and a thumb on each hand; and, although every voice has an individual quality about it, almost everyone can speak. These similarities and differences apply to every aspect of the body and mind. The physician's task, therefore, in making a diagnosis when John Smith is ill, is not to decide how his heart or lungs are different from Bill Brown's, but how his heart or lungs (or liver or leg or anything else) differ from what they are like when he is in good health, that is when the body and mind are working properly.

dent nurses watching an operation in a modern theatre; note the clothing.

There are many ways in which the physician can set about this, but principally he is dependent on two things: firstly what the patient can tell him and, secondly, what he can discover for himself by examining the patient. The first of these has not perhaps changed much in very many thousand years, except in so far as physicians have learnt what questions to ask, but the examination of the patient has changed enormously.

Physicians have always had their five senses. They can see, hear, touch, smell and taste. Of these, taste is the least important; except perhaps for tasting sugar in the urine of a diabetic, it has never been important in diagnosis. But they have always used the other four to help them to make a diagnosis.

Although the practitioner of today has no better faculties than practitioners of the past, his knowledge has been and still is increasing, so that the significance of what he can see and hear, feel and smell, is greater.

Thus although, as we have seen, even the ancient Egyptians knew that the heart spoke through the limbs, and the Chinese attached great importance to the pulse, it is only in the last two centuries that the pulse rate has come to be used as a significant measurement of the state of health or disease of the circulation and thus the body generally. For this it was necessary to have some accurate measure of short periods of time.

Sanctorius investigated the pulse rate in the early seventeenth century. At first he used a simple pendulum, adjusting the length of the string until it oscillated at the same rate as the pulse, using the length of the pendulum as the measure. Later he invented a primitive watch. Although a number of physicians investigated and wrote about the pulse rate in the next hundred years, it was not until the mid-eighteenth century that it became a regular part of the examination of the patient.

At about the same time, the practice of taking the patient's temperature began to be used. It had been observed from very early times that in certain illnesses the patient developed a fever, that is, became hot, but until the invention of the thermometer there was no means of measuring this with accuracy. Sanctorius attempted to measure temperature using a primitive form of thermometer. This worked on the principle that the air in a leaden bulb expanded and forced fluid along a marked column when it was warmed by being put in the mouth or under the arm.

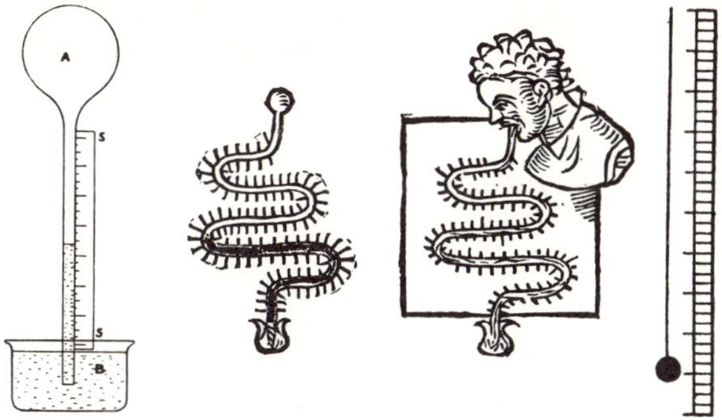

Early thermometers and pulsimeter

The invention of the mercury thermometer and the work done on it by Fahrenheit soon led to the development of an instrument which could reasonably be used in medical practice and such thermometers were available in England from 1740 onwards. It was not, however, for about another hundred years that the real value of temperature reading and recording was to be appreciated. Because the temperature of the body is altered in very many diseases, and because it changes rapidly and frequently in many cases, a great deal of work had to be done before the significance of its variation could be understood. When it is further realized that some of the early thermometers were nine inches or more long, took perhaps twenty minutes to reach the final temperature and had to be read without being removed from the patient's body, it is understandable that their full value was not at once appreciated.

Carl Wunderlich, in Leipzig, was the great pioneer in this work. He kept records of the temperatures of some twenty-five thousand patients and published the results in 1868.

In 1867 Dr Allbutt (later Sir Clifford Allbutt) designed and had made the first practical clinical thermometer for regular routine use.

> I wanted a thermometer which should live habitually in my pocket, and be as constantly with me, or more constantly, than a stethoscope. . . . It is scarcely six inches in length, and being slipped into a strong case not much thicker than a stout pencil, is carried in the pocket easily and safely . . .

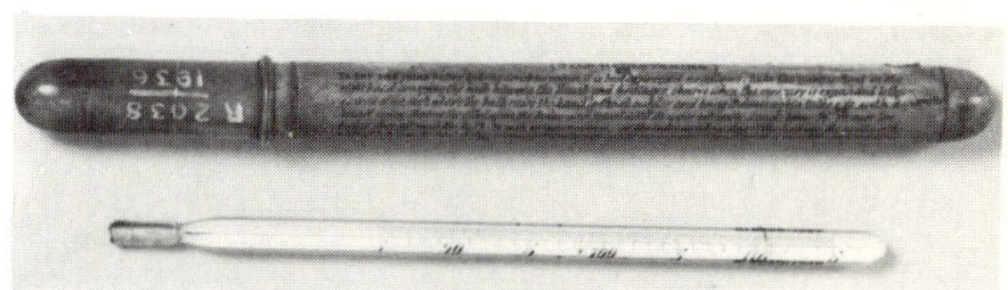

Thermometer as designed by Albutt, c. 1870

Although the thermometer and watch are an essential part of almost every medical practitioner's equipment today, it is the stethoscope which is most usually recognized as the inevitable accompaniment of the doctor. The stethoscope is an excellent example of how physicians have learned to make better use of their own senses. In this case, it is no more than a hollow tube which can be applied closely to the patient's body to enable the physician to hear better what noises are going on inside the patient.

Hippocrates had been well aware of learning by listening to noises within the body.

> You shall know by this that the chest contains water and not pus, if in applying the ear during a certain time on the side you perceive a noise like that of boiling vinegar.

In the middle of the eighteenth century Auenbrugger in Vienna described the sounds that could be heard on tapping the chest wall (percussion) and half a century later, in 1819, René Laennec in Paris wrote:

> . . . Taking a sheaf of paper I rolled it into a very tight roll, one end of which I placed over the praecordial region, whilst I put my ear to the other. I was both surprised and gratified at being able to hear the beating of the heart with much greater clearness and distinction than I had ever done before by direct application of my ear . . .

Following this, Laennec devised a wooden tube that would fit at one end against the patient's chest and at the other against his own ear. From Laennec's original stethoscope has developed the modern stethoscope and it can now be obtained with electronic amplifying devices inside.

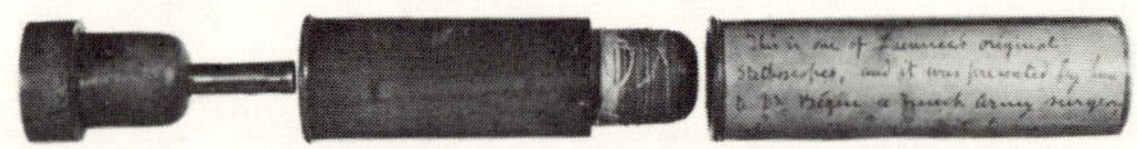

One of Laennec's original stethoscopes, partially dismantled

Great changes in methods of examination have been brought about by the development of mechanical and scientific devices that can be used to aid the physician's own senses. Magnifying lenses and microscopes are used in innumerable ways to see structures that are far, far too small to be seen with the unaided eye. Instruments have been devised with which to see into almost all the cavities within the body that can be reached by narrow, rigid tubes. In very recent years, with the development of fibre-optics, very slim tubes have been developed which can be passed into distant cavities in the body enabling the physician to see round many corners. With microcameras and electronic flashes, pictures can be taken deep inside the body.

Not only has modern science enabled the physician of today to see further and hear better within the body, it has added further 'senses' to the physician. As already mentioned, the human body is an extremely complicated working machine and much of its working is controlled by minute electrical currents. With appropriate apparatus these electrical currents can be detected and, amplified many times, can be made to trace graphs on paper. From this has come the electrocardiograph and electroencephalograph which enable the electric currents generated within the heart and brain to be recorded, and abnormalities to be detected when no other method would reveal anything amiss.

There are many other developments enabling more and more to be discovered about the workings of the body both in health and in disease. Most of these (with the exception of X-rays which are dealt with in Chapter Ten) are too recent for their place in medical history to be even guessed at as yet.

When the diagnosis has been made, with or without the assistance of modern apparatus, there remains the problem of treatment, of what help to give the patient. Over the years, that help has varied and expanded enormously. It is perhaps relevant here to indicate how the mechanical apparatus to provide that help has expanded. The early flint knives and wooden splints of prehistory have led to the exceedingly complicated apparatus of a modern operating theatre. Much could be said about progressive developments, especially in the operating theatre, but space does not permit this. However, the illustration of the heart-lung machine shown overleaf may give some idea of the increase in the complexity of the equipment used directly and indirectly in surgical procedures.

It is an example of the apparatus used in operating theatres today. For minutes, or even hours at a time, the machine does the work of the patient's heart in circulating the blood when the heart has been stopped for an operation on it. It also does much of the work of the patient's lungs when breathing has also been stopped.

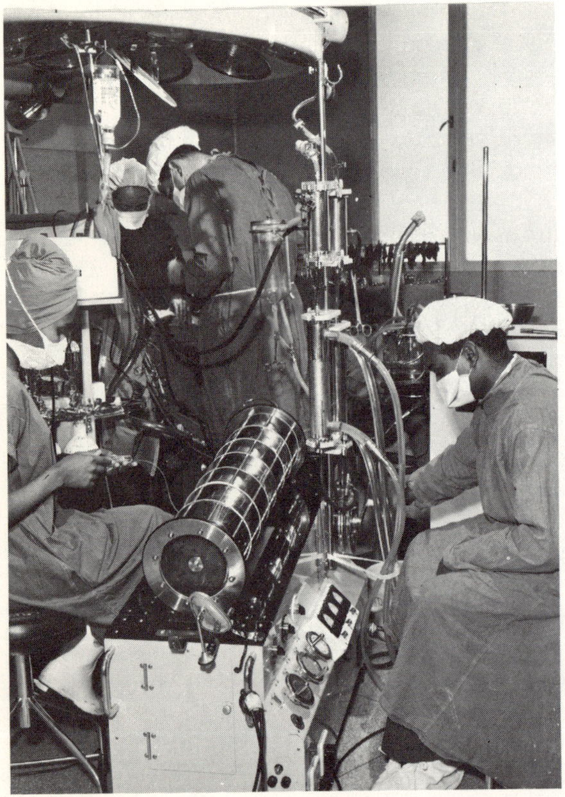

The Melrose heart-lung machine in use at the Hammersmith Hospital, London

It is impossible to say how many people are involved in modern operations. There might indeed be only six or eight people in the operating theatre, but dozens and perhaps hundreds of people are involved indirectly. The surgeon, the anaesthetist and the theatre sister are essential people but they need the help of those who have designed and built the theatre and all the apparatus used, the doctors, nurses and technicians who have done the investigations beforehand and those who will look after the patient during his recovery. In addition, there is everyone who makes the hospital work, without whom the operating theatre could hardly be used.

Despite all these remarkable advances, and the great advances in treatment that will be mentioned later, everything ultimately depends on man. There is not yet, nor will there ever be, a magic to solve the problems of disease. There are only men devoting their labours to the task of helping their fellows. However complicated and mystical medicine might seem to be, medicine is only a form of help towards regaining or retaining health. In the final analysis, it is always the patient who must achieve that health for himself however great the help that is given might be.

CHAPTER SEVEN
More and more science

We have already seen how the progress of medicine has depended on discoveries and advances in fields of learning far removed from medicine. We have seen how the work of Vesalius became much more widely known and understood because of the invention of printing than it would otherwise have been: how the work of Harvey needed the invention of the microscope to show how the blood completed its passage from arteries to veins through the capillaries: how an understanding of the significance of pulse rate and temperature depended on the invention of watches and thermometers.

During the seventeenth and eighteenth centuries many fields of scientific thought and investigation had been developing. Physics and chemistry had been freed from mediaeval ideas and the strict control of the churchmen and a new understanding of the subjects was developed. Galileo and Newton had revolutionized physics, Robert Boyle had changed alchemy into chemistry. Oxygen was discovered and shown to be the part of air essential for human life.

At the beginning of the seventeenth century astrology, the influence of the planets and stars on human life, was widely considered of use in diagnosis and prognosis, but before the end of the eighteenth century it had no place at all.

Throughout this time the newly acquired knowledge was considered in relation to medicine and causes of disease. Ideas and theories based on investigation and reason sought to explain the nature and origins of disease. There was perhaps a risk in this rapidly developing scientific understanding of the processes of nature that, to the medical practitioner, the new knowledge would become more important than his patient, and that risk is still present today.

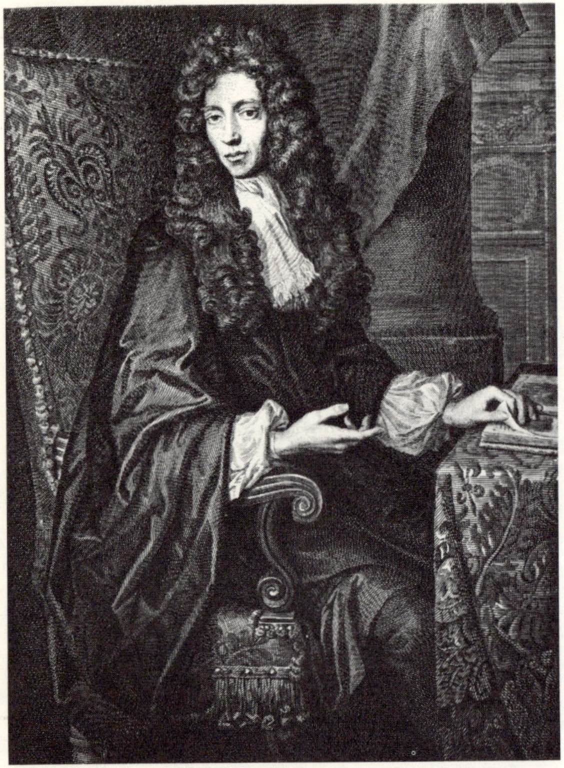

Engraving of Robert Boyle (1627–1691) prefixed to an eighteenth century edition of his writings

Two men, however, deserve special mention for doing much to keep the well-being of the patient as the principal purpose of medical practice, but who, at the same time, encouraged observation and reasoned thinking as the basis of progress. These are Thomas Sydenham, a physician in England in the seventeenth century, and Hermann Boerhaave, who practised at Leyden in Holland from the beginning of the eighteenth century. Sydenham believed that the best place to learn about illness was at the bedside, observing the natural course of disease, and the way to help the patient was not to treat him unnecessarily. Writing about scarlet fever he says:

> . . . By treatment thus simple and natural, their ailment – we can hardly call it more – is dispelled without either trouble or danger: whereas, if, on the other hand, we overtreat the patient by confining him to his bed, or by throwing in cordials, and other superfluous and over-learned medicines, the disease is aggravated, and the sick man dies of his doctor . . .

Sydenham's writings guided English physicians for very many years and not without reason has he been called the 'English Hippocrates'. He died in 1689.

The importance of Boerhaave's influence on medical practice cannot perhaps be overstated. He made no great medical discoveries but he was sympathetic to new ideas and when convinced of their value he was prepared to use them in his practice. When he was appointed Professor of Botany and Medicine at Leyden in 1701 he instituted the method of teaching that has become accepted throughout the world in medical schools. Instead of confining his lectures to the classroom he demonstrated the symptoms and signs of disease at the bedside. If the patient died he made a post-mortem examination and demonstrated to his students the disease processes inside the body that had given rise to the signs and symptoms in life. This he did long before post-mortem examinations were usual practice.

He was considered to be the greatest medical teacher of his century and he drew students from all over the world to study under him. His pupils, full of the enthusiasm that he had inspired, carried his ideas and methods to far places. When the medical school was founded at Edinburgh in 1726 many of its first professors were one time students of Boerhaave's.

At this time, and indeed until the medical department of the College of Philadelphia was opened in 1765, there was no medical school in America. Many Americans came to Europe to study medicine and especially to Edinburgh and Leyden. Thus did Boerhaave's teachings cross the Atlantic. So much so that in 1760, in the city in which the first medical school was to be opened five years later, a Dr Rush wrote:

> . . . The system of Dr Boerhaave governed the practice of every physician in Philadelphia . . .

It is not perhaps surprising that the story is told of how a letter addressed simply to 'The Greatest Physician in the World' was delivered to him. Another version of the same story is that he received a letter from China addressed simply 'Dr Boerhaave – Europe'.

Men such as these kept medicine firmly centred on the patient as a human being but, with the coming of the nineteenth century, science came more and more to the fore.

We have already learnt that anatomy is the science of the structure of the body and physiology the science of how the body works. Disease is the result of something going wrong with the proper harmony of the

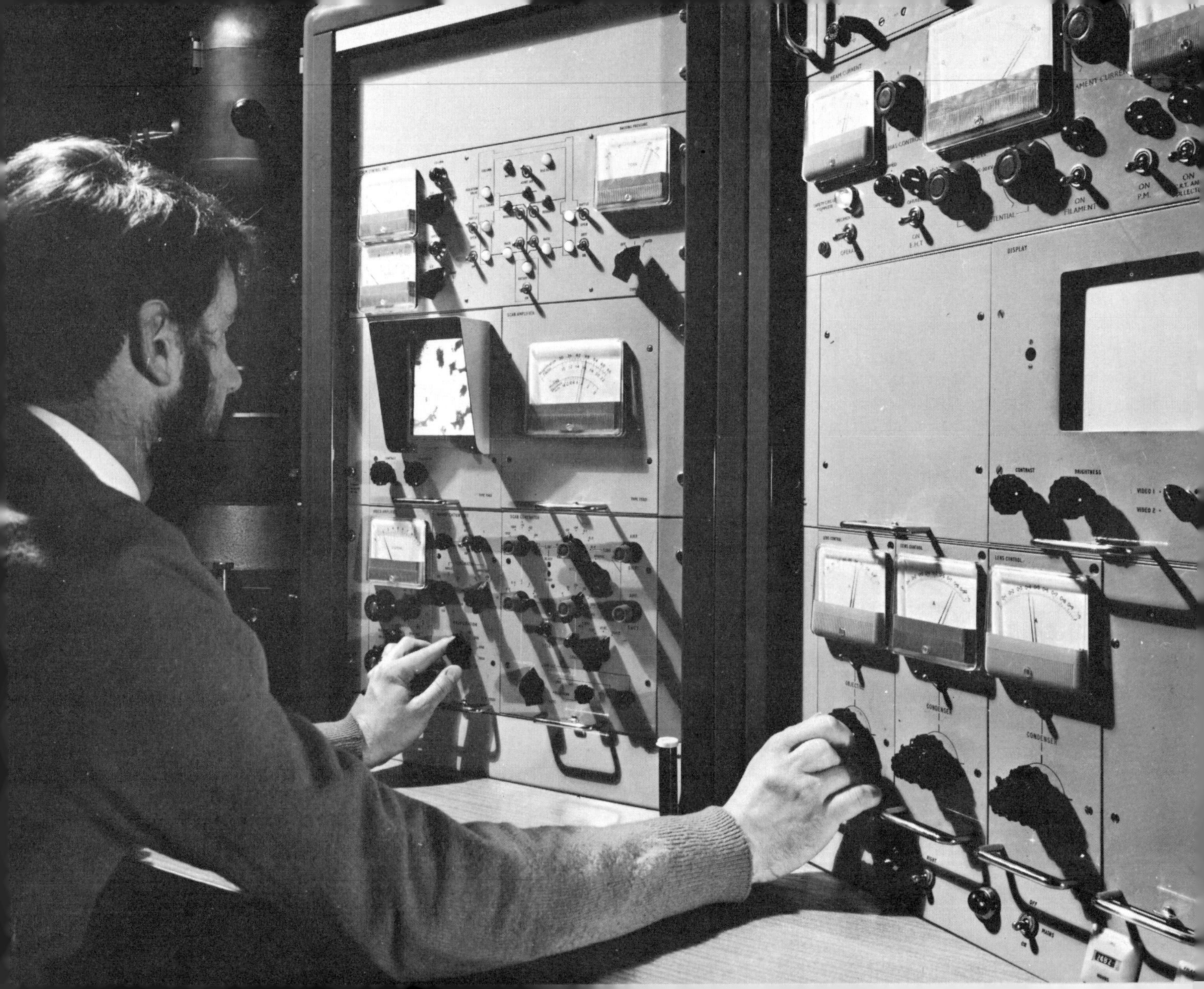
BEAM CURRENT
ON
P.M.
ON
FILAMENT
ON
E.H.T
DISPLAY
CONTRAST
BRIGHTNESS
VIDEO 1
VIDEO 2
SCAN AMPLIFIER
LENS CONTROL
CONDENSER
CONDENSER
OFF
MAINS

body and pathology is the name given to the science of disease and disease processes. We have seen how disease was originally thought to be a punishment from the gods. This gave place to the humoral theory of the Greeks in which disease was regarded as an imbalance of the humours. Further progress on the nature of disease could not develop, however, until a proper understanding of anatomy and physiology had begun, for one cannot tell what is abnormal unless one knows what the normal should be.

One of the great obstacles to the study of anatomy was the objection to post-mortem dissection and examination. This was perhaps an even greater hindrance to the development of pathology because it was not a question of finding *a* body to dissect but in examining post-mortem a *particular body* that had suffered from a particular disease. It came, however, to be accepted that only through detailed post-mortem examinations could disease be fully understood.

Giovanni Morgagni of Padua in 1761 published an important book of pathological examinations, but Matthew Baillie, a Scotsman in England, in 1793 was the first to treat pathology as a systematic study.

The further developments of pathology were, as we have seen in other fields, dependent on improvements in fields of knowledge outside medicine. The microscope came to be much improved beyond the simple instruments of van Leeuwenhoek and, as the nineteenth century advanced, better and better descriptions of tissues were made. In 1858 Rudolph Virchow of Berlin established the fundamental principle of pathology that the basic unit of all animal tissue whether healthy or diseased is the cell: that a cell can only arise from another cell and that no living tissue can come from anything other than a cell.

Further refinements of methods have continued to give more and more information and today, with the electron microscope illustrated opposite, smaller and smaller structures can be seen. It still remains true that cells can only develop from cells, but now the anatomy of the cell is perhaps almost as complicated as was the anatomy of the whole body when Vesalius first described it.

With the growth of pathology various branches of the subject have gradually appeared and themselves given rise to further divisions. Louis Pasteur (see also Chapters

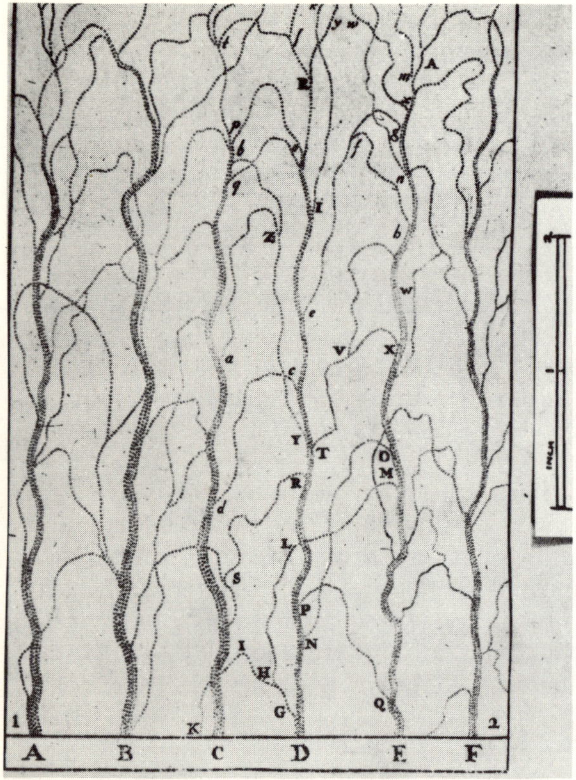

A diagram by van Leeuwenhoek which shows the capillary network in the web of a frog's foot

Eight and Twelve) who disproved the idea of spontaneous generation of bacteria, showed that germs only arise from germs much as Virchow showed that cells only arise from cells. He, and Robert Koch in Germany, who discovered the tubercle bacillus, created the branch of pathology known as bacteriology, the study of germs, from which in turn has further developed virology. Viruses are living organisms so small that they can only be seen with electron microscopes, yet they are the cause of many of the common infectious illnesses such as measles, mumps, chicken-pox and the common cold.

Another important branch of pathology is the study of the blood, or haematology. From the days when the first red blood corpuscle was seen possibly by van Leeuwenhoek, to the present, our understanding has developed enormously. The number of red cells in the blood (about five million per cubic millimetre or twenty-five thousand million in a teaspoonful) was first reliably counted in 1852 and the white cells recognized three years later – there being about one white cell for every thousand red cells.

Almost all doctors in practice today will have memories of the laborious process of counting hundreds of cells in measured and diluted volumes of blood to determine whether or not patients had normal numbers. Today it is done in seconds by electronic counting devices.

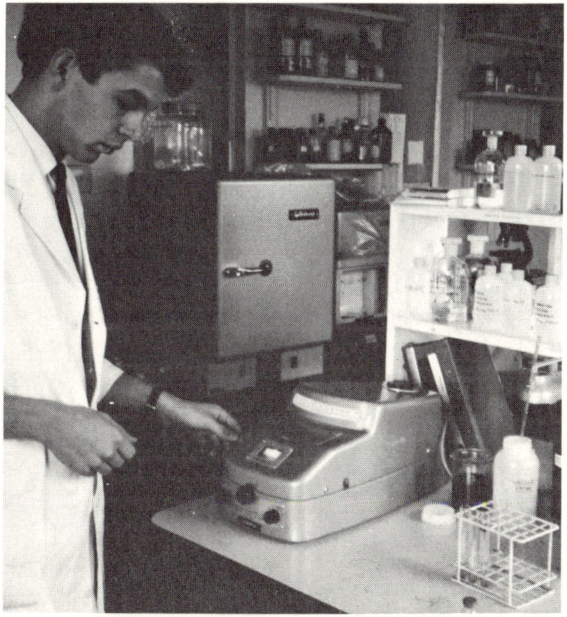

Technician using a modern colorimeter in the biochemical department of a modern pathology laboratory

In the middle of the nineteenth century biochemistry, the chemistry of living organisms and the substances associated with them, and chemical pathology, the chemistry of disease processes, also began to be developed. This in turn has grown until, in the present automated and computer age, there are automatic laboratories where from one specimen of blood a dozen or more estimations of the chemicals in it can be obtained. In minutes procedures are carried out which would have taken a technician several hours to perform only a few years ago.

Thus is the process of examination and diagnosis becoming more and more detailed and scientific. The benefits that may come from this are great, but so also are the dangers. As more and more knowledge of the human body and how it works is discovered it is becoming possible for doctors to forestall disease before there is any 'dis-ease' at all. In Chapter Eleven in particular we shall consider the progress of treatment. Treatment depends on diagnosis. Whereas at the beginning of the scientific era there was little known and not much of material benefit to do, today so much can be done that it is easy to forget the healing power of nature.

CHAPTER EIGHT
Setting the stage for modern surgery

Surgical operations are so commonplace today that many of those reading these words will themselves have undergone an operation for some reason or another. There will be very few indeed who do not know someone who has had an operation.

Although operations are often performed to save life, they are also today undertaken for much less than life-saving reasons and few people are terrified by the prospect of an operation even on themselves. This, however, has not always been the case and in our present civilization it is really only in the last hundred years that surgery has been looked upon as anything other than a last resort.

Today one not only hears of operations to save life being undertaken on the heart and the brain for instance which take many hours (four, six or even eight-hour operations are not unknown), but also of operations which are performed for cosmetic reasons alone without there being any need for surgery at all other than alterations in the individual's appearance. This has almost all come about in the last century and much of it in the last half-century or less.

Although we have already encountered (in the first chapter of this book) evidence of certain operations which were performed many thousands of years ago, there were three major obstacles to any real progress in surgery until quite recent times. These were *bleeding*, *pain* and *infection*.

It is perhaps natural enough that a good deal of the early (and some of the later) progress of surgery should have come as the result of injuries sustained on the battlefield, for it is there that large numbers of injuries occur. Indeed, surgery consists largely of dealing with wounds and it is only because surgeons have learnt how to deal with wounds that they are able to make wounds in the right places and in the right ways, thus enabling them to correct troubles within the body. The illustration opposite is taken from a sixteenth century surgical handbook and indicates the types of wounds with which a surgeon might have had to deal.

The first of the great advances in operating was established by Ambroïse Paré, one of the humblest, but also one of the greatest, of surgeons more than four hundred years ago. Ambroïse Paré was a French surgeon who gained much of his early experience through treating soldiers wounded on the battlefield and it was Paré who first popularized the method of stopping bleeding by ligation (tying a thread round the bleeding vessels) rather than cauterizing with a red-hot iron. A red-hot iron does indeed stop the bleeding but, as can well be imagined, it is desperately painful and, of course, also causes much damage to tissues. Ligation had certainly been used at times in the past but it was not until Paré came on the scene that it was established as the best and proper method to use.

At the beginning of the sixteenth century, when Paré was a young man, it was believed that all gunshot wounds were poisoned and the poison must be burnt out with boiling

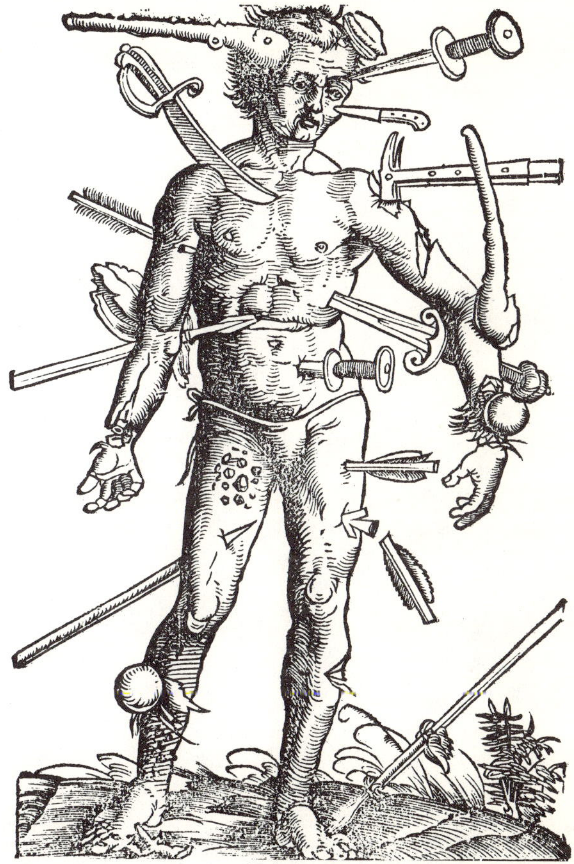

A woundman from a German surgical handbook, 1530

oil. However, following one battle in 1536, there were so many casualties that the supply of boiling oil was exhausted.

> . . . Now because there were some few left to be dressed, I was forced, that I might seem to want nothing, and that I might not leave them undressed, to apply a digestive [a poultice] made of the yolk of an egg, oyle of Roses, and Turpentine. I could not sleep all that night, for I was troubled in mind, and the dressings of the precedent day, (which I judged unfit) troubled my thoughts. . . . Therefore I rose early in the morning. I visited my patients and beyond expectation, I found such as I had dressed with a digestive onely, free of vehemencie of paine to have had good rests, and that their wounds were not inflamed, nor tumifyed: but on the contrary the others that were burnt with the scalding oyle were feverish, tormented with much paine, and the parts about their wounds were swolne. When I had many times tryed this in divers others I thought this much, that neither I nor any other should ever cauterize any wounded with Gun-shot.

It was perhaps this experience in his early life as a surgeon, for he was only twenty-six at the time, or one similar that induced in him the great humility expressed in his works so often. 'I dressed the wounds – God healed them.' Instead of using the drastic measures so often practised to cure patients he realized that the less the natural healing processes of the body were interfered with, the better the result.

Despite this advance and despite the great advances in the knowledge of the structure and functions of the human body following on the work of Vesalius in the same century and William Harvey in the next (see Chapter Five), it was not until the middle of the nineteenth century that the next great obstacle to surgery was overcome. This was the discovery of effective anaesthesia.

Before 1846 the most important attribute needed by a surgeon was speed. Surgical operations by their very nature were bound to be painful and the quicker the operation the less time there was to suffer pain. Nor was this only a matter of the patient's comfort, for pain produces shock and shock itself can kill. Thus, not only would patients be very reluctant to undergo operations lasting more than a very short time, but also, if surgeons did take longer than necessary, they increased the chance of killing the patient however successful the operation itself might be.

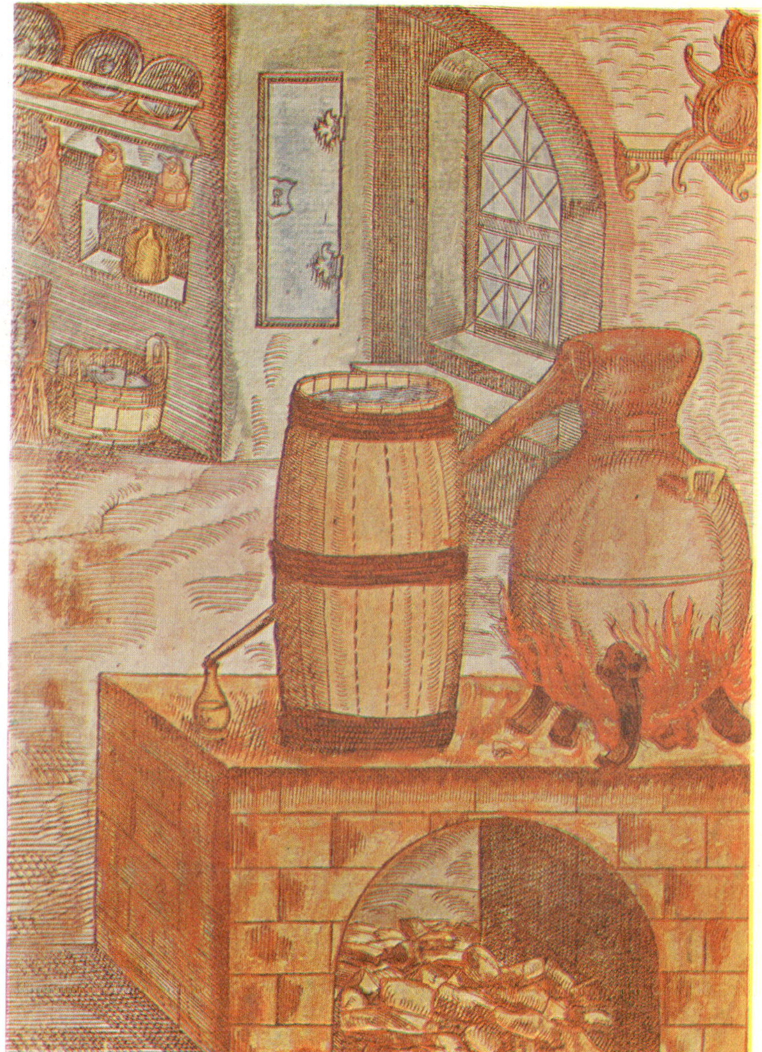

Book illustration of a sixteenth century laboratory; a liquid is being distilled. Compare the apparatus with that in the pathology laboratory on page 45.

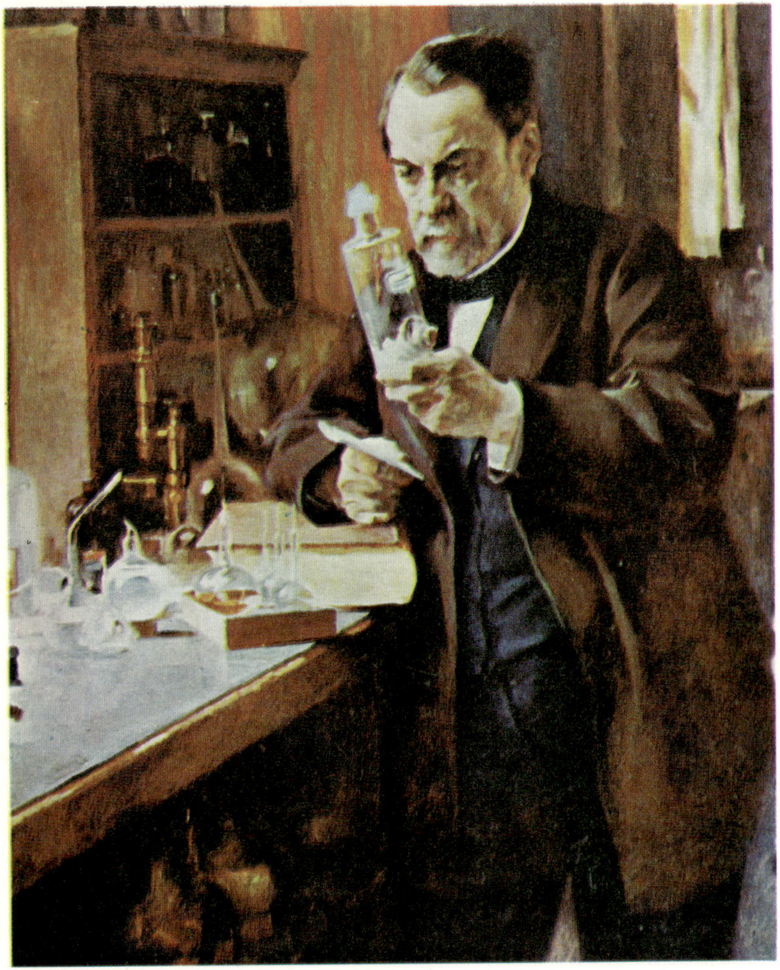

Louis Pasteur in his laboratory in 1885; the wisp of cotton wool in the glass vessel he is examining is to prevent germs contamining the contents.

As an example of the speed that was necessary, William Cheselden, who died in 1752, was reputed to have perfected the operation of lithotomy (cutting for stone in the bladder) to such an extent that he had completed the operation in fifty-four seconds. Moreover he had reduced the mortality rate of this operation to seven per cent.

This need for speed, however, severely limited the type of operation that could be attempted. Amputations of limbs, the removal of superficial tumours, cutting for stone, these were the usual type of operations.

We have seen that major operations had taken place even in the very distant past and certainly some diminution of pain could be obtained by the use of drugs such as opium and alcohol. It may be that drugs to prevent pain were known and used in ancient civilizations of which all trace has now been lost. In Peru the Coca bush grows, and from this bush has been extracted cocaine. It may be that the Incas of Peru used this as an anaesthetic long before Columbus discovered the New World. We have no written evidence of this for the Incas had no system of writing, but we do know from relics that have been found that they did perform quite major surgery.

Another form of anaesthetic, the significance of which might be greater than we know, is that of hypnosis or mesmerism. James Esdaile, when working as a surgeon for the East India Company, performed two hundred and sixty-one operations in India using mesmerism, but when he retired to Scotland found that the Scottish patients did not respond to his methods. As modern anaesthetics were discovered about this time, the need for mesmerism disappeared.

Laughing-gas (nitrous oxide) and ether were both discovered some time before this and were used occasionally at parties as intoxicants. Sir Humphrey Davy had tried inhaling laughing-gas and even suggested its use for surgery, but it was not until 1842 that a surgical operation was performed under an inhaled anaesthetic. This was the removal of a small tumour from the neck of a Mr Venable, under the influence of ether, by Crawford Williamson Long in America.

> . . . I commenced inhaling the ether before the operation was commenced and continued it until the operation was over. I did not feel the slightest pain from the operation and could not believe the tumour was removed until it was shown to me . . .

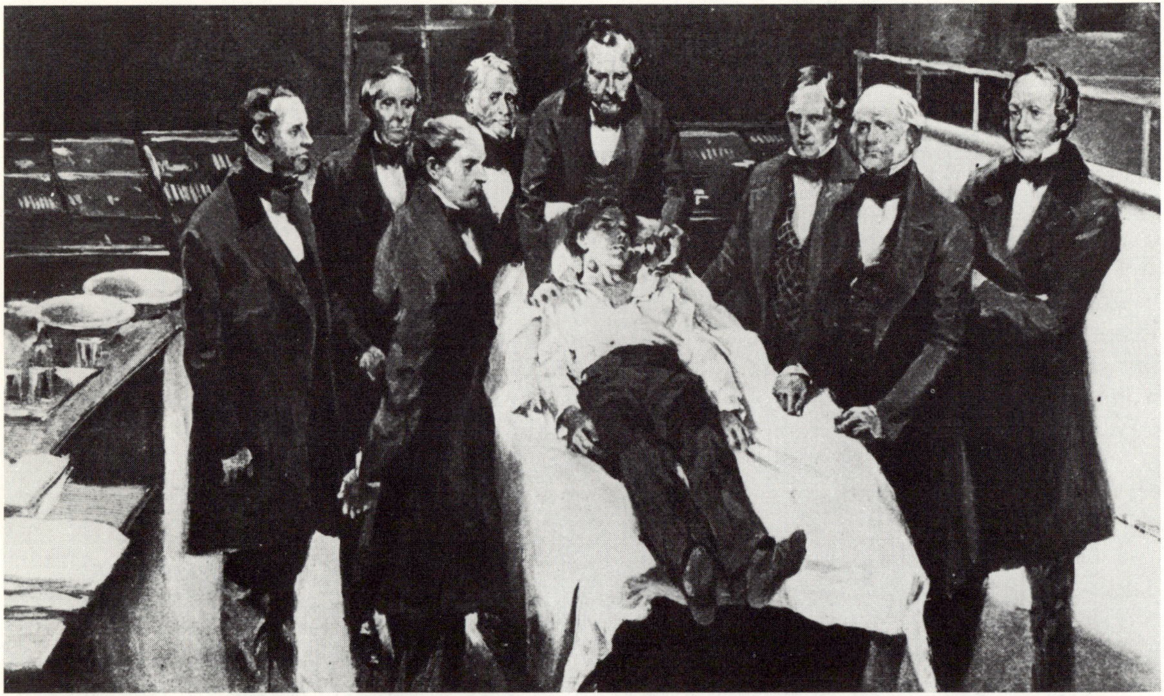

The first public demonstration of surgical anaesthesia in Boston, U.S.A.

In the next few years occasional operations, mostly for extracting teeth, were performed whilst the patient was under the effects of nitrous oxide or ether. The first published information was of an operation in the Massachusetts General Hospital, Boston, on 16th October 1846 under ether anaesthesia. Within a month it was being used in Britain.

By January 1847, however, chloroform had been used for the same purpose by Sir James Young Simpson in Edinburgh and within a short time it was in general use throughout the world. Chloroform had several advantages over ether in that it was easier and pleasanter to use both for the surgeon and the patient, a much smaller quantity was necessary and it was not explosive. The illustration on this page shows diagrammatically the workings of a very early type of chloroform inhaler and may be compared with the picture of modern anaesthetic apparatus shown on page 55. Since the middle of the nineteenth century, however, many different anaesthetic agents have been discovered and today anaesthesia is a highly specialized and complicated technique. It has come a long way from merely taking the pain away from an operation.

Many modern operations, such as those on the heart and lungs, depend as much on the skills of the anaesthetists as on the surgeons themselves. In these operations it may be necessary temporarily to stop the heart and lungs working. The circulation and respiration are then maintained artificially by the anaesthetist and a number of assistants.

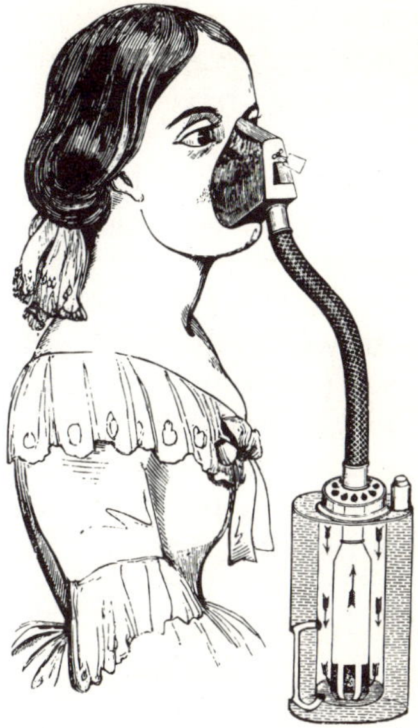

John Snow's chloroform inhaler, 1858

So far only general anaesthesia has been considered, that is making the patient unconscious. Towards the end of the nineteenth century, however, a substance, which had some years earlier been purified from the coca plant of Peru and called cocaine, was found to cause local insensitivity to pain when applied in solution to the eye and other parts of the body. It was soon also used by injection under the skin for minor operations. Since then other local anaesthetics have been developed and used extensively for minor operations on the surface of the body. They can also be used under certain conditions for some quite major operations.

With the discovery and development of effective anaesthesia, however, the third great obstacle to surgery had still to be overcome: that of infection. The fact that inflammation and pus formation almost always occurred in surgical wounds was accepted as natural and even desirable until the nature of infection began to be understood. Inflammation and pus formation are indeed natural in that they are the means whereby the body fights infection. Inflammation is caused by the tissues of the body preparing to fight invading germs, and pus consists mainly of innumerable millions of white cells which the body brings to the scene of 'invasion' and which attempt to destroy the invading germs.

Before 1864 inflammation was thought to arise spontaneously in wounds, although there had been one or two men with an inkling of the true nature of the problem. About the end of the eighteenth century two British obstetricians (specialists concerned with childbirth), Dr Gordon of Aberdeen and Dr White of Manchester both suggested that puerperal fever was contagious and Gordon said clearly that it was carried from patient to patient by midwives and physicians. In America in 1843, Oliver Wendell Holmes, in an essay, said that obstetricians should not take part in post-mortems on puerperal fever victims. His advice was, however, unheeded.

At about this time a Viennese obstetrician, Ignaz Phillip Semmelweiss, realized that patients attended by students, who also attended post-mortems, were more frequently the victims of puerperal fever than patients attended by midwives, who did not attend post-mortems. He realized that in some way this disease could be conveyed by uncleanliness and, in 1861, wrote:

> . . . The carrier of the decomposed animal organic material is the examining finger, the operating hand, the bedclothes, the atmospheric air, sponges, the hands of midwives and nurses . . .
>
> . . . A proof of this is that before the introduction of chlorine disinfection nearly all the patients . . . (who were examined in a particular manner) . . . died of puerperal fever.

At this time the true nature of infection was not understood even though, as with Semmelweiss, some measures had been found helpful in preventing it. It was not, however, to be long before the foundations of understanding were to be laid.

In 1864, Louis Pasteur a French chemist who had been working on the problems of fermentation in wines, finally proved that infection was in all cases due to germs, some of which were carried in fine particles in the air.

> . . . There is now no circumstance known in which it can be confirmed that microscopic beings have come into the world without germs, without parents similar to themselves. Those who maintain these views are victims of illusions, of ill conducted experiments, blighted with errors that they have either been unable to perceive or unable to avoid.

In the following year, Joseph Lister, a surgeon in Glasgow, having read of Pasteur's work realized its significance for surgery and the antiseptic era of surgery had begun.

Before this time it had been believed generally that putrefaction was due to the oxygen or other gases in the air. Lister realized that it was not the gases in the air but germs suspended in the air which caused the putrefaction.

> . . . Turning now to the question how the atmosphere produces decomposition of organic substances, we find that a flood of light has been thrown upon this most important subject by the philosophic researches of M. Pasteur . . .
>
> . . . In the course of the year 1864 I was much struck with an account of the remarkable effects produced by carbolic acid upon the sewage of the town of Carlisle . . .
>
> . . . My attention having for several years been much directed to the subject of suppuration . . . the applicability of carbolic acid for the treatment of compound fracture naturally occurred to me.
>
> My first attempt of this kind was made in the Glasgow Royal Infirmary in March 1865. . . . It proved unsuccessful, in consequence, as I now believe, of improper management; but subsequent trials have more than realized my most sanguine anticipations.
>
> Case 1. James G— aged 11 years, was admitted into the Glasgow Royal Infirmary on 12th August 1865 with compound fracture of the left leg, caused by the wheel of an empty cart passing over the limb. . . My house surgeon Dr Macfee, acting under my instructions,

laid a piece of lint dipped in liquid carbolic acid upon the wound. . . . It was left undisturbed for four days . . . I now dressed the wound with lint with water having a small proportion of carbolic acid diffused through it: . . . this was continued for five days . . . I substituted for it a solution of one part carbolic acid in from ten to twenty parts of olive oil, . . . At the expiration of six weeks I examined the condition of the bones, and, finding them firmly united, discarded the splints; and two days later the sore was entirely healed, . . .

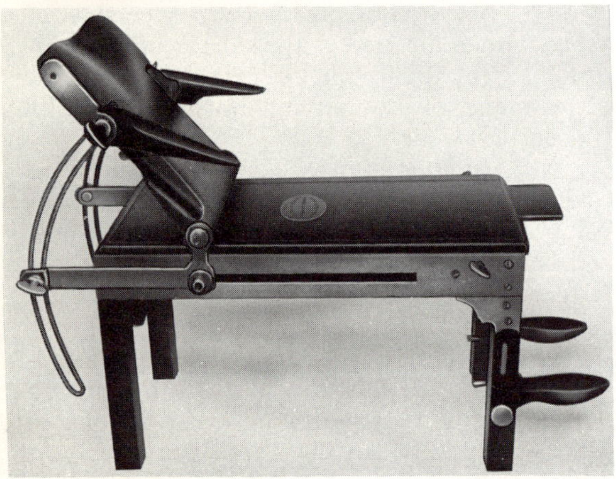

Operating table used by Lister

For many years after this, Lister pioneered the method of antisepsis in surgery. One method of dealing with the germs in the atmosphere was to have a fine spray of carbolic acid in a cloud over and around the operation site. The illustration facing page forty-eight shows how a typical operation scene would have looked. The figure on the right of the picture is directing the carbolic acid spray (sometimes hand pumped but here steam operated) towards the operation site. The spray was not liked by Lister, nor the other surgeons who used it, but it was indeed a most important step towards the surgery of today. There was at first much scepticism, especially in London whence he came after leaving Glasgow. In 1877 Lister remarked,

> I wonder how long it will be before the truth is recognized by English surgeons! If it is the truth, gentlemen, the time will come.

Gradually his principles were accepted and, in his lifetime, he was recognized as one of the great men of surgery.

In many other ways Lister aided the progress of surgery although he will be remembered chiefly for his work in connection with antisepsis. Another valuable achievement

Modern operating theatre, Boston, Engl

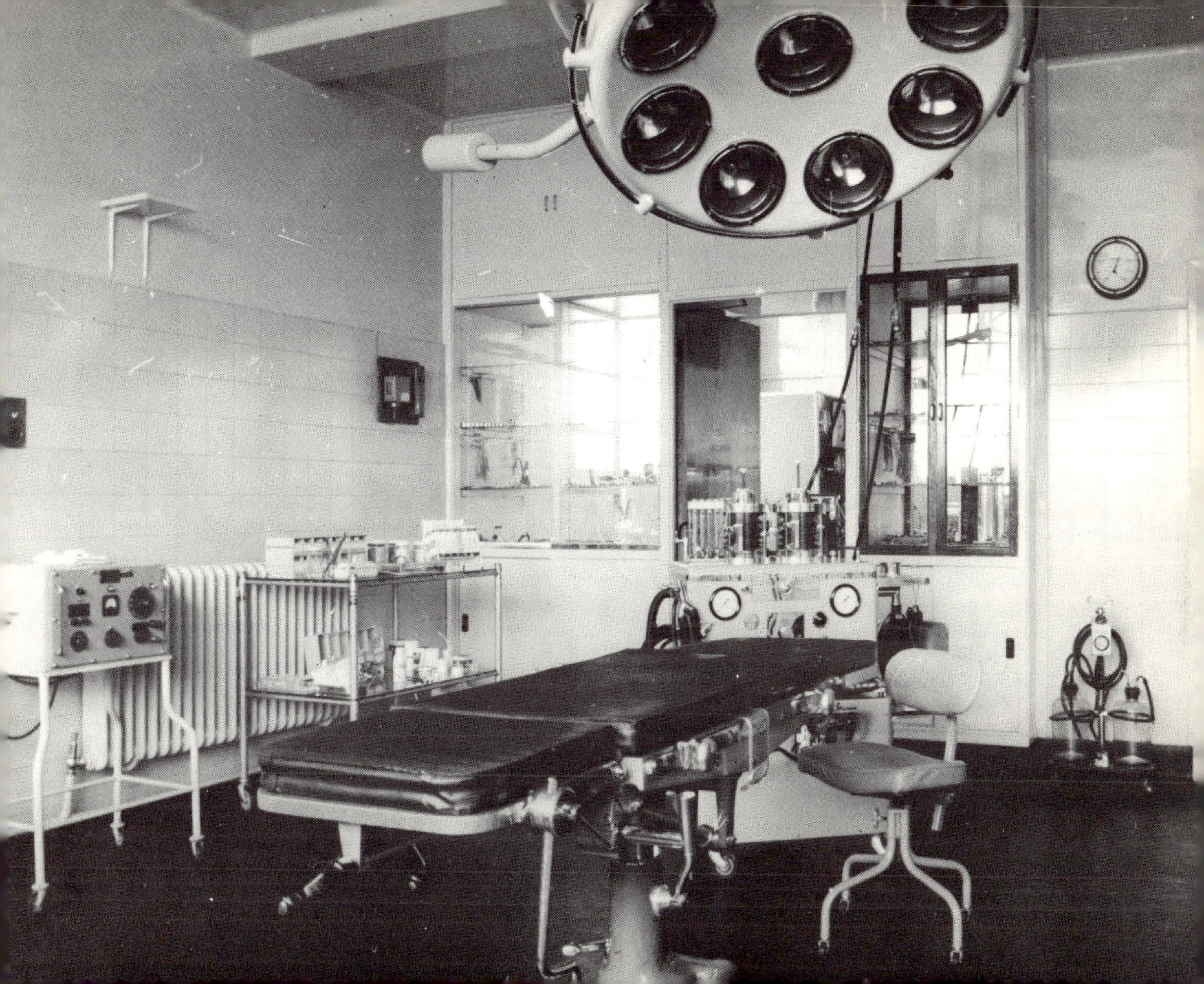

was his discovery of the use of catgut as a suture material. He found that this could be used for ligatures and stitches inside the body and eventually would be absorbed.

At this time, as the illustrations show, Joseph Lister and his disciples, as well as all other surgeons, used to operate in their ordinary clothes, often in ordinary rooms. They did not perhaps use their walking-out suits, but this was because they did not want their good clothes spoiled by blood and not because of the germs that they carried.

From the 1870s onwards, however, the methods of dealing with infection have been both by keeping infection away from surgical wounds by asepsis and by killing any germs that do infect the wound by antisepsis.

Nowadays, as almost everyone will know, the hands and clothing of a surgeon and everyone else in an operating theatre are, so far as possible, cleansed of germs before they approach the patient. All the instruments, dressings and even the air in the theatre are made as germ free as possible. If, despite this, germs do contaminate wounds, and this does sometimes happen, antiseptic methods are used. Nowadays this is more usually by chemotherapeutic and antibiotic substances such as sulphonamides and penicillin than by carbolic acid. But the principle of killing the germs without harming the tissues of the patient is the same.

Without these steps the lengthy, and sometimes enormously complicated operations of today would not have been possible, as all the efforts of the surgeons would have been destroyed by infecting germs.

Today surgery has many subdivisions. Within the abdomen it developed rapidly, especially from the work of Billroth in Vienna. Theodor Kocher in Switzerland contributed enormously, especially to the surgery of the thyroid gland, and was the first surgeon to receive a Nobel Prize (1909). Surgery within the chest, hindered by the need for sub-atmospheric pressure in the thorax to maintain respiration, was pioneered by Sauerbruck. Today the patient's respiration is controlled by the anaesthetist, leading in turn to the development of cardiac surgery. Neurosurgery has grown in the last half century and now no part of the body is beyond the potential help of surgery.

Although beyond anything imaginable even a century ago today's complexities could not have come without the pioneers.

CHAPTER NINE
Mental illness

When a man has a wound it can be seen and from one's own experience it is fairly easy to understand something of the pain that he might be suffering and the disability that he might have. If a leg is broken there is no difficulty in understanding why the injury prevents walking, nor with an arm the corresponding problems.

If a disease is not visible but the patient is of sound mind, he can describe and explain his troubles and one can understand at least what the patient is saying.

If, however, the mind is ill, what the patient says and does is far less easy to understand. If a man's actions are not based on reason then ordinary people, whose actions are based on reason, may have great difficulty in understanding why he acts as he does.

If a man stands petrified in front of a lion, or runs away and cowers in a corner, his action is understandable. If, however, the lion is not really there, the man's actions are inexplicable unless one knows that he has imagined that he saw a lion. Suppose, however, that he struck out at the imaginary lion with a hatchet or spear. This would be reasonable if there really was a lion but terribly dangerous for everyone else if there were no lion and the man was imagining lions everywhere.

Mental illness is a disorder of the mind and, in some way, the power of reasoning is affected. This is usually in less obvious ways than having hallucinations, the name given to seeing or hearing things which are not really there, but it always means in some way that the patient's actions are unreasonable.

Mental illness has been recognized from very early times. For a long time mental illness was regarded as due to 'being possessed by a devil' and the treatment was to drive out the devil by a variety of methods.

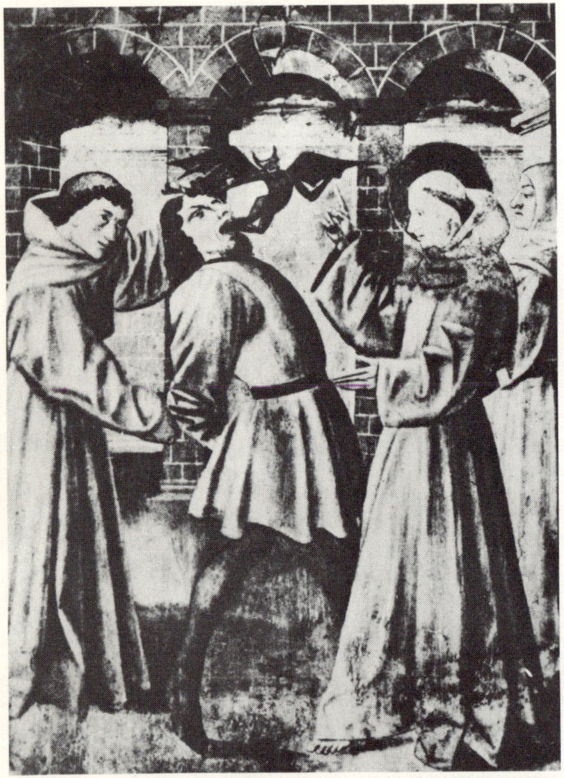

Italian fresco which shows St Antony of Padua casting out a devil

It came to be believed that anyone possessed of a devil, that is mentally ill, should be destroyed. Unfortunately the Church gave official approval to this in the fifth century. It was not, however, until the late Middle Ages that the great witch hunts took place, which resulted in many thousands of innocent people being put horribly to death.

As early as the first century AD Soranus of Ephesus, a Greek physician, described many forms of mental illness and recommended methods of treatment that were based on kindness and humanity. Despite this, over the centuries, lack of understanding, and fear caused by the irrational actions of some mentally ill people, made the usual method of dealing with them to have them put away and locked up so that they could do no harm.

In lunatic asylums it was usual to chain up many patients and they were treated like wild animals. Bethlem Hospital (Bedlam) in London first received lunatics in 1377. In about 1400 its equipment included 'manacles, chains of iron, locks and keys and stocks'.

Although in isolated instances in the years from 1500 to 1800 a few physicians did make attempts to study and help mental illness, no real progress was made. The best that could be hoped for was that patients in asylums would be fed and not ill-treated too violently. The illustration opposite shows how, in fact, they were often restrained. In this case the patient was chained to the walls of his cell.

The first real changes came independently of one another in the Bicêtre Hospital in Paris and in building the Retreat in York.

In 1791 one Hannah Mills, a Quaker, died in the Lunatic Asylum at York. Permission had been refused for friends to visit her. As a direct result of this, William Tuke and other members of the Society of Friends investigated the possibility of raising money and building a hospital.

> At a Meeting of Friends held at York the 28th of 6th month, 1792, for the purpose of taking into consideration the propriety of providing a retired Habitation, with necessary advice, attendance, Etc., for the Members of our Society, and others in profession with us, who may be in a state of Lunacy, or so deranged in mind as to require such a provision,
>
> RESOLVED
>
> that persons of this description, (who are truly objects of great sympathy and compassion) . . . and the feelings of their near connexions are rendered more dissatisfied and uncomfortable

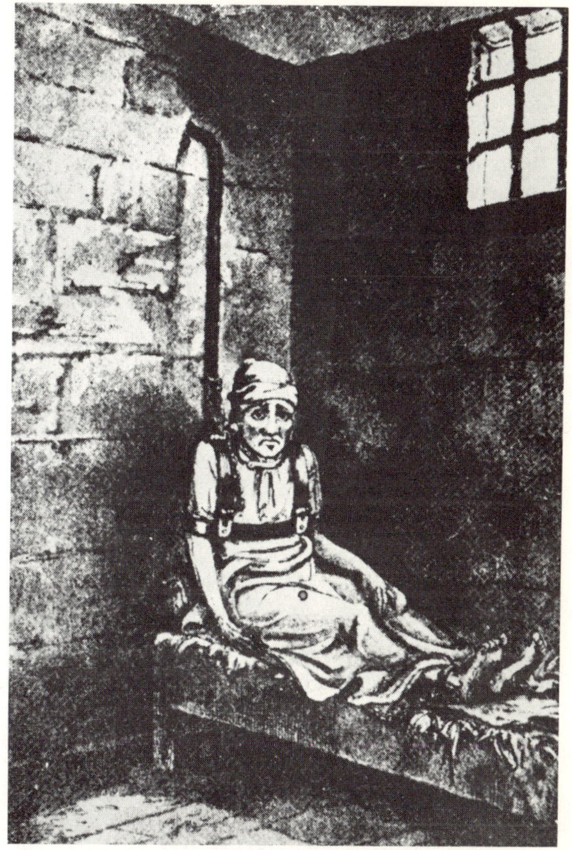

Nineteenth century drawing of a mental patient

> than would probably be the case, if they were under the notice and care of those, with whom they are connected in Religious Society. It appears, therefore, very desirable that an Institution should be formed. . . . This would, doubtless, in some degree, alleviate the anxiety of the relatives, render the minds of the Patients more easy in their lucid intervals, and consequently tend to facilitate and promote their recovery . . .

In 1794 the building was begun and patients were admitted either at the end of 1795 or early in 1796. This building was called, and is still named, the Retreat. It was the first hospital in the world to be built specifically with the intention of treating persons suffering from mental illness with as little restraint and as much consideration as possible.

At almost the same time as building began on the Retreat at York, Philippe Pinel in Paris was appointed as physician superintendent of the Asylum de Bicêtre. There he found one man who had been confined for forty years and another who had been in chains for thirty-six years. The conditions were appalling. He believed that such restraint was unnecessary and after much difficulty he finally obtained permission from the National Assembly to remove the chains in 1798. This he did, despite opposition, and to the surprise of many people the patients responded to the kindness shown them.

These two events, the building of the Retreat at York by William Tuke and the striking off of the chains in the Bicêtre by Philippe Pinel, were the beginnings of a completely changed attitude to mental illness. They were, however, only the beginning and it was to be many years yet before the same attitude would be general in all asylums.

One of the earliest asylums to adopt the practice of abolishing physical restraint was the Lincoln Lunatic Asylum where, following the appointment of Dr Robert Gardiner Hill, restraint was rapidly reduced as the table opposite shows.

In 1839, at Hanwell, England, Dr Conolly, another pioneer in the treatment of mental illness, abolished mechanical restraint and a few years later wrote that there was:

> no asylum in the world in which mechanical restraint may not be abolished not only with safety, but with incalculable advantage.

Conditions improved over the succeeding years and laws were passed controlling the conditions in all mental hospitals.

Year	Total Number of Patients in the house	Total Number of Patients Restrained	Total Number of Instances of Restraint	Total Number of hours passed under Restraint
1829	72	39	1727	20,424
1830	92	54	2364	27,113¾
1831	70	40	1004	10,830
1832	81	55	1401	15,671½
1833	87	44	1109	12,003½
1834	109	45	647	6,597
1835	108	28	323	2,874
1836	115	12	39	334
1837	130	2	3	28
1838	148	0	0	0

Table of restraint at Lincoln Lunatic Asylum where Dr. Gardiner Hill (house surgeon from 1835 to 1838) advocated and showed the possibility of total abolition of physical restraint.

Philippe Pinel, in addition to his humanitarian attitude, also laid much of the foundation of the real understanding of mental disease.

> . . . I, therefore, resolved to adopt that method of investigation which has invariably succeeded in all the departments of natural history, viz. to notice successively every fact, without any other object than that of collecting material for future use; and to endeavour, as far as possible, to divest myself of the influence, both of my own prepossessions and the authority of others . . .

This is a similar attitude of mind to that which we have already seen in Hippocrates, in Paré and in Vesalius. These men did not disregard what others had done and said, but they were determined to discover for themselves, where possible, what was the truth. Only by such methods are the mistakes of the past put right and thereby fresh knowledge discovered.

Progress in the real understanding of mental illness was to be slow for the next hundred years, but progress there was to be.

The writings of Sigmund Freud, Alfred Adler and Carl Jung, men who have done much of their work in the present twentieth century, are especially important as they have contributed a great deal to the understanding of the workings of the subconscious and unconscious mind.

With the beginnings of the understanding of the mind, treatment has also begun to be possible. Electro-convulsive treatment (ECT) as a means of treating some illnesses where the patient becomes unreasonably depressed, and some other forms of illness, has only been in use since 1934. It is even more recently, only in the 1950s, that effective drugs have been discovered, and are still being discovered, to help illnesses where mania and schizophrenia are the main trouble. The benefits of these drugs, however, are already sufficiently apparent to have justified the research necessary for their development.

These advances are all too recent to have any real place as yet in history. Much work remains to be done, but the philosophy of Hippocrates, that all illness is a natural phenomenon and not a supernatural one, and the determination to observe, observe and observe again, to treat with kindness and to help nature but not to interfere unnecessarily as shown by Pinel, is still the basis of real progress for the future.

CHAPTER TEN
X-rays and radioactivity

Whenever men practise medicine, one of their most important functions is to make a diagnosis, to decide the cause of the patient's illness.

A diagnosis, however, is not always a complete identification of the patient's illness, but the more exact and complete it is the more exact and complete the treatment can be. If a man has a pain in his chest it is a diagnosis, though only a very incomplete one, to say that he has 'a pain in the chest'. It is obviously desirable to know much more about its cause because the treatment to help a disease of the heart would not be the same as that for pneumonia in the lungs. Neither treatment would be the same as that for a broken rib.

As we have already seen, doctors have continually tried to find better and better methods of discovering just what has been wrong with their patients. We have already seen how such instruments as thermometers and stethoscopes have been developed in order to find out more precisely what was wrong. Man has always had his eyes but, until 1895, he could only use those to see the surface of the body, or into cavities such as the mouth and ear, unless a cut was made to expose the inside of some parts of the body. However, in 1895, Wilhelm Conrad Röntgen discovered what he called X-rays and what have come to be known throughout the world by that name.

Professor Röntgen was a physicist and not a doctor. The first public announcement of his discovery was on 28th December 1895, when he read a paper *On a New Kind of Rays* before the Wurzburg Society in Germany.

> . . . We soon discover that all bodies are transparent to this agent, though in very different degrees. I proceed to give a few examples: paper is very transparent; behind a bound book of about one thousand pages I saw the fluorescent screen light up brightly. . . . If the hand

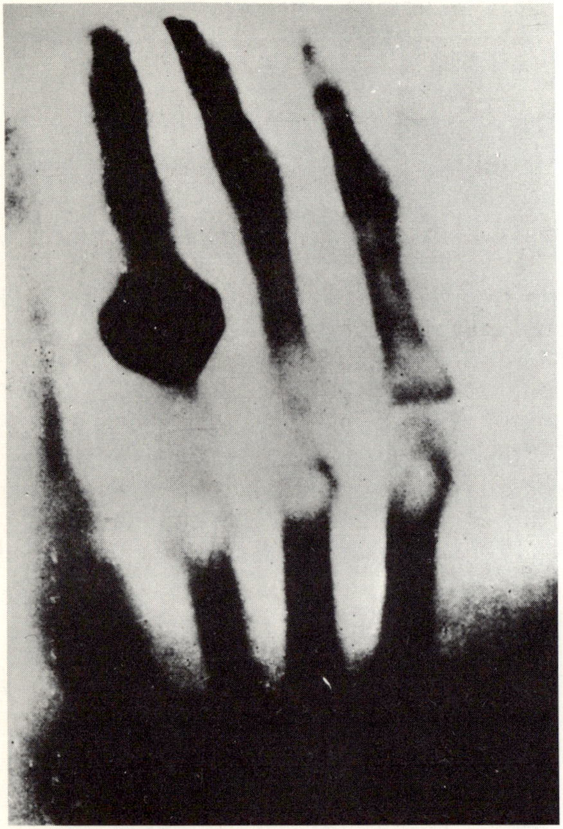

X-ray of Rontgen's wife's hand, December, 1895

be held between the discharge tube and the screen, the darker shadow of the bones is seen within the slightly dark shadow-image of the hand itself . . .

The illustration is of an X-ray picture made by Rontgen of his wife's hand on 22nd December 1895. It is probably the first X-ray picture of human tissues ever taken.

Although some of those present at that meeting might have foreseen something of the value of the new discovery to medicine, no one could have guessed the enormous value, nor the dangers, that would come from it. Within a very few years X-ray machines were to be found in all the larger cities of the world and nowadays, little more than seventy years later, hardly a hospital in the civilized world is without its X-ray apparatus.

In 1895, for the first time, it was possible to see something of what was inside the human body without cutting a hole to look.

X-rays, however, only cast shadows of radio-opaque materials and it is only because bone is more radio-opaque than other tissues in the body that X-ray (shadow) pictures can be taken of them. It is not possible to take X-ray pictures of many of the other tissues of the body but it was not long before it was

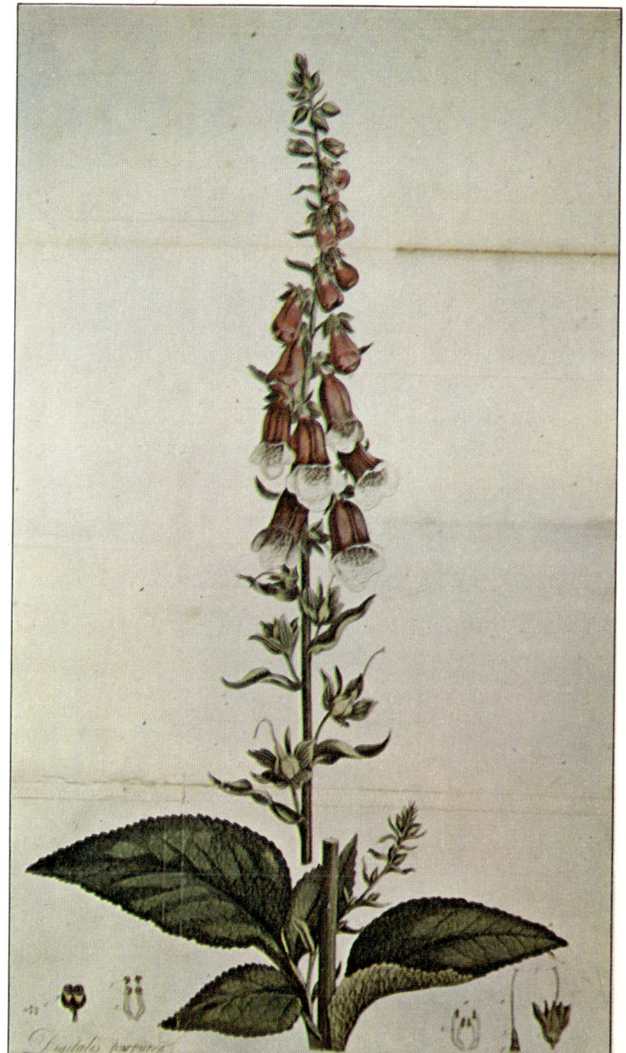

An illustration from William Withering's 'An Account of the Foxglove', *1785; the lower section shows the parts of the plant used for certain heart diseases.*

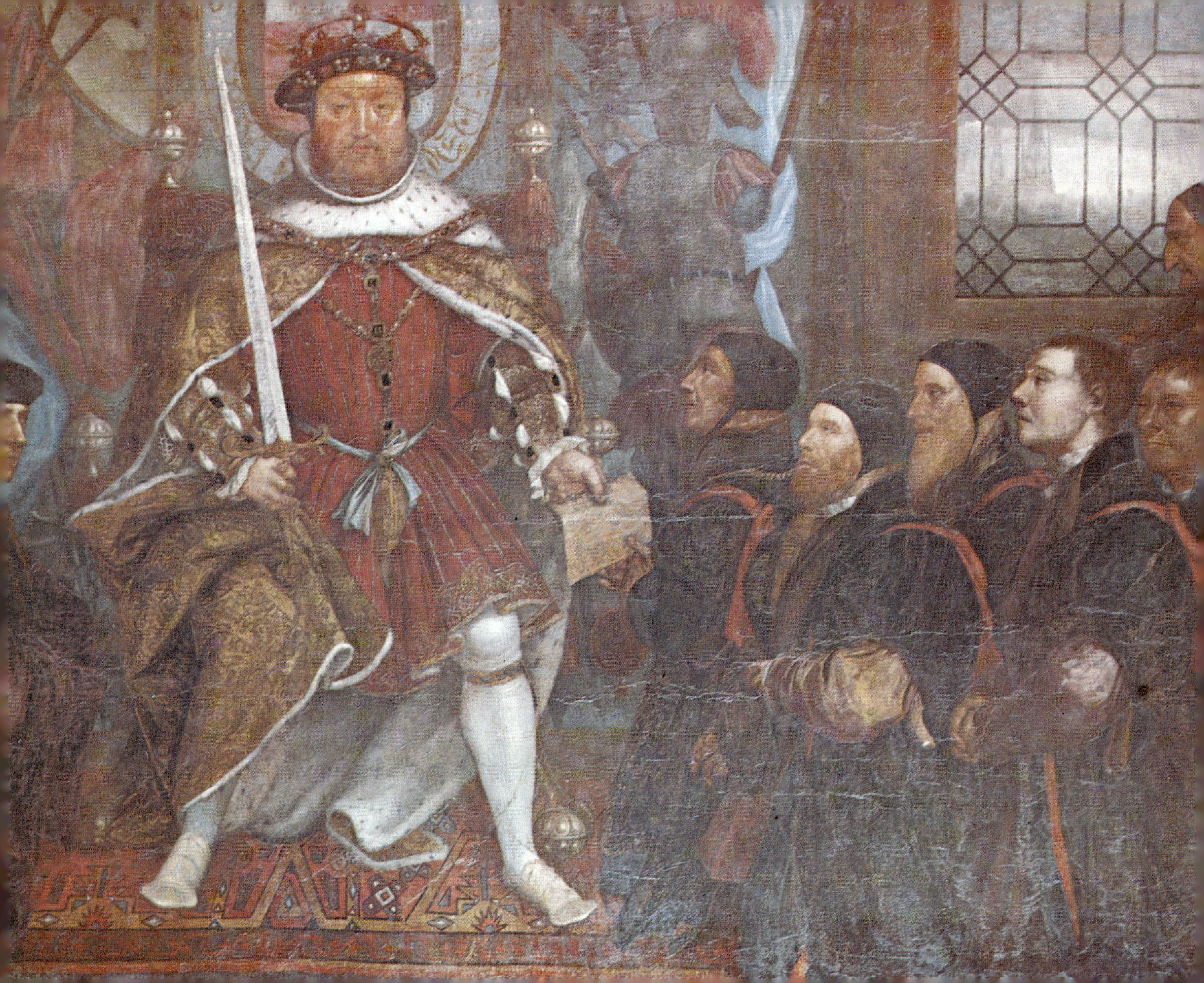

realized that if hollow organs, such as the stomach, could be filled with radio-opaque substances X-rays could be taken to show the outline of the cavity that had been filled.

Barium salts (which soon replaced the Bismuth salts used initially) were made into thick gruel like soups and, after they had been swallowed by patients, X-rays showing the outlines of their stomachs and intestines could be taken. Although not as good as seeing directly it was very much more informative than not being able to see anything at all.

Since then, by numerous technical processes, ways and means have been discovered whereby it is possible to take X-ray pictures of almost every space inside the body. Pictures of the tubes in the kidneys and the liver, of the air tubes in the lungs, of blood vessels throughout the body and even the fluid-filled spaces inside the brain, all can be shown more or less well on an X-ray shadow picture.

When X-rays began to be used, it was not immediately realized that they had certain dangers and many early workers suffered severe and even fatal injuries. The slowness in recognizing the dangers was due to the fact that the effect is not immediate and that repeated doses of X-rays are cumulative in effect. (This can perhaps be better understood by comparing it with sunlight and sunburn, the effects of which, however, are not so long delayed.)

The realization that continued or repeated exposure to X-rays affected the tissues of the body led to two important developments which have been, and are still being, pursued. These are the development of methods which would protect both operator and patient from unnecessary exposure to the X-rays, and the development of radiotherapy (treatment by radiation).

The necessity of protecting both the patient and the operator from the ill effects of the rays was especially important for the operator because, although the patient would be fully exposed to the rays on one or two occasions, the operator would be present and indirectly exposed innumerable times. This has led through many stages until now it is possible for the radiologist to watch by means of television, and moving picture X-rays of patients can be stored on video-tape for repeated examination without repeated exposure to radiation and, if desired, they can be seen by many people. Of course, X-ray still pictures (which is all that is necessary for

·nry VIII conferring the Act of Union on the barbers and surgeons in 1540.

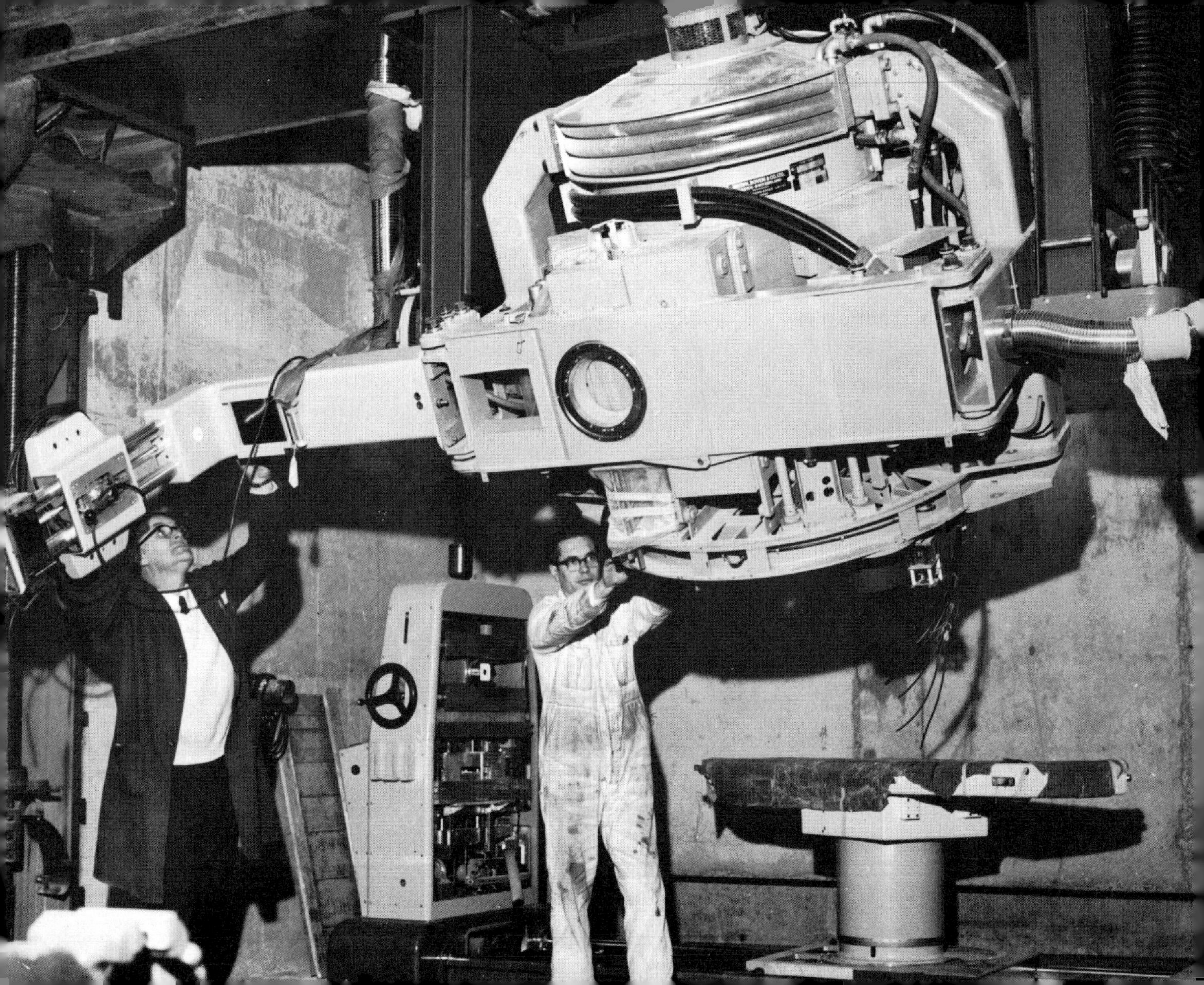

most bone and joint X-rays) have always been stored and available, but it is only very recently indeed that the picture on the X-ray screen, for investigations such as Barium meals, could be seen by more than one or two people for a fleeting moment of time.

The fact that X-rays affected the tissues through which they passed led to the development of radiotherapy which is now a major branch of medical practice.

Within a year or two of their discovery, X-rays had been used to treat some skin diseases. With the discovery of natural radiation by Becquerel and the subsequent discovery of radium by Pierre and Marie Curie, which followed many years of hard and painstaking work in primitive conditions in Paris, the real history of radiotherapy began. The first one-tenth of a gramme of pure radium was produced in 1902 from many tons of pitch-blende. In the previous year Pierre Curie had confirmed Henri Becquerel's findings that radiation could burn living tissues.

For their work on radiation phenomena Becquerel and the two Curies were awarded the Nobel Prize for Physics in 1903. With this came international recognition but only

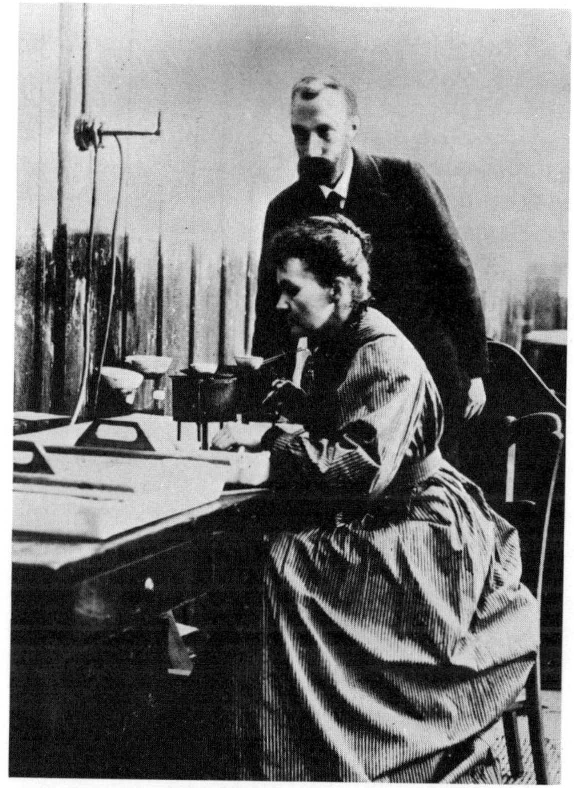

Pierre and Marie Curie at work together in their laboratory

ain's most powerful radiotherapeutic equipment at Guildford

three years later Pierre was killed in a street accident. Nevertheless, Marie continued the work, conducted the world's only course for students on radioactivity, and in 1911 was again awarded the Nobel Prize, this time in Chemistry, for her work on the chemistry of radioactive elements.

From the time of the discovery of radium until relatively recent years, radiotherapy offered the only alternative to surgery in the treatment of cancer. Often it was the only treatment. Today other drugs and methods are proving of great use but radiotherapy remains a principal treatment. It has progressed enormously until today when extremely costly and very powerful sources of radiation are used. This form of treatment is confined to a few specialized units because of cost and the highly specialized staff needed. The more powerful units such as the thirty-five million electron volt betatron at Guildford need housing in special radiation-proof concrete and lead glass rooms to prevent radiation escaping to the outside world.

Progress in this branch of medicine has, in recent years, been much more rapid than it might otherwise have been because of the vast military and industrial research going on in electronics and radiation and many other branches of medicine have been helped by developments in nuclear physics. The ability to make certain elements radioactive has helped medical research greatly. When an element is made radioactive and included in something taken into the body, either as food or as an injection, the course that the element takes in the body can be followed. This is done by a Geiger counter showing whereabouts in the body the element is. This has enabled scientists to discover much more about how the body works than they could have discovered in any other way and it is being of use both in diagnosis and in some cases in treatment of disease.

An example of this is to be found in the diagnosis, and sometimes in the treatment, of certain forms of disease of the thyroid gland in the neck. The thyroid gland uses iodine and, if a measured dose of radioactive iodine is taken by the patient the radioactivity over this gland can be measured. This enables it to be seen whether the gland is working properly or not.

The full potential of this type of tool in the treatment of disease remains to be seen and is not for a present 'history of medicine'.

CHAPTER ELEVEN
Therapeutics

Therapeutics is the branch of medicine concerned with the uses of drugs and medicines, but really it covers all forms of treatment.

Therapy, or treatment, has always involved advice to the patient on how to conduct his life and in either doing something to or for him, or giving him a medicine to take.

Human nature being what it is, and probably not having changed much in thousands of years, men have hoped for magic to cure their ills. They have not found magic but, in turning to medical practitioners they have found men, and more recently women, genuinely anxious to provide help. This is perhaps the one constant and unchanged aspect of medical practice since it first began.

The advice and treatment offered by the good physician has always depended on his understanding of the nature and the cause of the disease and his knowledge of available methods of treatment.

When disease was believed to be sent by the gods it was natural enough for sacrifices to be offered to the gods. These would most naturally have come to be offered through the intermediacy of the priest. In turn, this would have led to the priests of the particular gods favoured for healing having frequent contact with sick people and thus increasing experience of illness and disease. Not only would they have acted as priests but also probably they would have incorporated advice gained by experience in their instructions to the patients. Thus, the treatment available from the priest-physicians of Egypt and Greece would have been likely to have included experienced advice as well as religious ministrations. We have already seen something of this in Chapters Two and Three.

But ideas regarding the causation of disease changed to belief in it being caused by the humours. When disease was thought to be

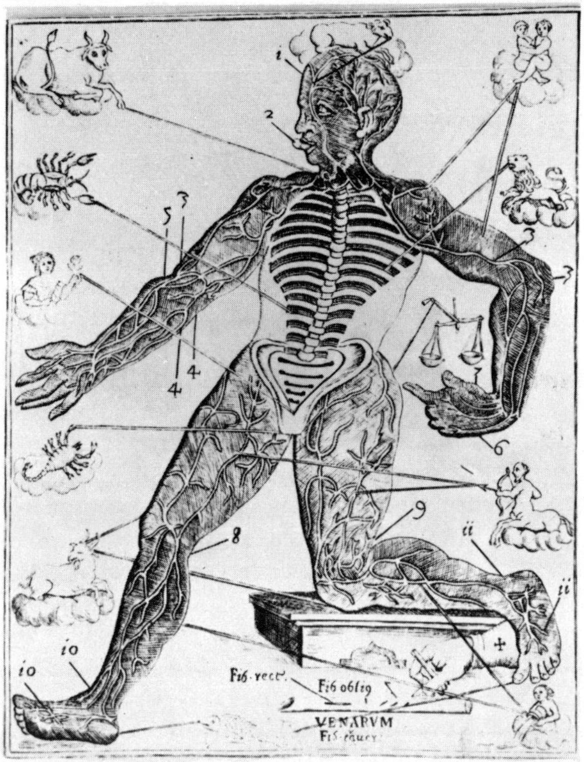

Diagram showing points where blood may be let

due to an excess of one of the humours – blood, phlegm, yellow bile and black bile – it was natural enough that physicians tried to improve matters by letting out the excess. As this was the accepted basis of disease from the time of Aristotle in the fourth century BC and continued to be for more than two thousand years, it is not surprising that blood letting, purging and vomiting were recommended and accepted treatments.

During much of this time another science played its part in medicine. Astrology (the influence of the stars on human activities) had been studied from very early times in Egypt and frequently treatment of disease was influenced by the patient's horoscope. It was believed that certain days were favourable or others particularly unfavourable for various treatments. Even as late as the eighteenth century Richard Mead, an eminent London physician and physician to Queen Anne, wrote a book, *A Treatise Concerning the Influence of the Sun and Moon on Human Bodies.*

In the early part of the sixteenth century an outspoken, and in many ways brilliant, man appeared on the scene. This was Philippus Theophrastus Auriolus Bombastus von Hohenheim, better known as Paracelcus.

Paracelcus, of Swiss-German origin, was born in 1493. He was perhaps the forerunner of modern therapuetics but he was born too early for his ideas to be acceptable or even understood. He travelled widely; in his early years searching for knowledge and gaining experience, and in his latter years trying to find an audience that would listen to him.

Whilst he was still a child his father was appointed municipal physician at Villach, where there were mines and a mining school, and he there gained a much greater knowledge of practical chemistry than was usual in physicians at that time. Throughout his life he emphasized the use of chemicals in medicine; he tried to use simple single substances in treatment rather than the very complicated prescriptions usual in those days, and among other chemicals he introduced mercury and iron to European therapeutics.

He built his practice of medicine on the sound foundations of his own experience and observation of nature: he searched for the effective principle in medicines and discarded the unnecessary and complicated and, as such, was perhaps the first scientific chemist in medicine; he attached considerable importance to astrology which to him probably signified the importance of taking into account the whole environment as the cause

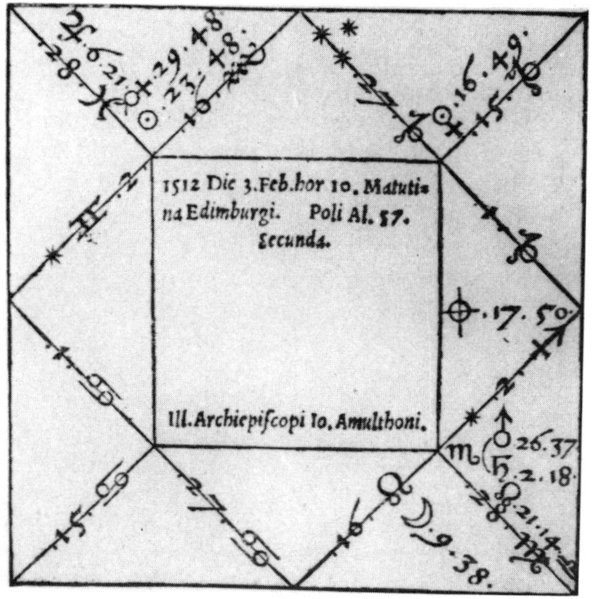

Horoscope of Archbishop Hamilton of St Andrew's, 1552

of disease: and, fourthly, he believed that the foundation of medical practice lay in love for one's fellow men.

Despite these sound principles he was not readily accepted in his lifetime: he was too outspoken and far from modest. Before

Vesalius had shown the errors of Galen in anatomy, Paracelcus publicly decried Galen and Avicenna and is supposed to have emphasized this by burning their books before beginning a course of lectures. He did not conform to the dress or manners of the profession of the time and he did not attempt to hide his scorn for whatever he regarded as foolish and wrong.

The first words of his ever to appear in print were in a pamphlet announcing his lectures at Basle. In it he wrote:

> . . . Who does not know that most doctors today make terrible mistakes, greatly to the harm of their patients? Who does not know that this is because they cling too anxiously to the teachings of Hippocrates, Galen, Avicenna and others?
>
> . . . Day after day I publicly elucidate for two hours . . . books written by myself. I did not, like other medical writers, compile these books out of extracts from Hippocrates or Galen, but in ceaseless toil I created them anew, upon the foundation of experience, the supreme teacher of all things . . .

It is hardly surprising that his ideas were not readily acceptable to the rest of his profession.

At this time, and indeed really until the last hundred years or so, treatment by medicines and drugs was almost wholly empirical. That is to say, medicines were used because experience had shown that they worked without the reasons for their effects being understood.

Strange and wonderful concoctions of medicines, against so many of which Paracelcus was so outspoken, were used until

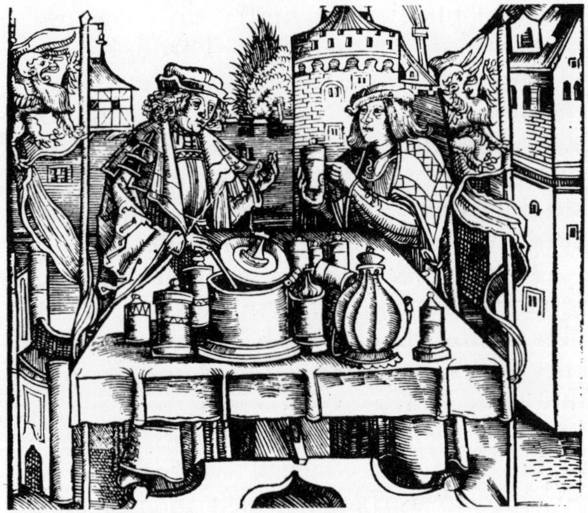

Ceremonial preparation of theriac in the early sixteenth century

quite recent times. Theriac is perhaps the most famous of these. It was believed to be an antidote against all poisons, bites and stings and to help both in the prevention and treatment of most diseases. The Roman Emperor Marcus Aurelius took a dose every day and it was certainly being used in England in the sixteenth century. Doubtless it started as a fairly simple prescription but over the years ingredients were added to improve it until ultimately it contained seventy-five different items. (Some such as opium and squills can be powerful drugs and might have beneficial effects.) It is unlikely that any ingredients were removed as people would fear that they were diminishing the efficacy of the medicine.

Until the eighteenth century there were very few specific remedies in the form of drugs. There were a few powerful drugs such as opium which had been used from very early times to relieve pain, and castor oil which was used as a purgative, but these, like most others, were symptomatic remedies in that they treated a symptom rather than the underlying cause of a particular disease. However, as diagnosis did not go much beyond the recognition of certain symptoms, perhaps the drugs did as much as was asked of them.

The science of pharmacology, the preparation and action of drugs, is an essential part of modern therapeutics. But, although the preparation of drugs began in the mists of prehistory, a scientific approach to therapeutics could hardly develop until pathology, physics and chemistry had been developed and their scientific principles been applied to medicine and the actions of drugs in and on the human being.

As a separate science in its own right pharmacology did not develop until the early nineteenth century, mainly in Germany, and in Britain only in the last quarter of that century. However, long before then the foundations were being laid.

One of the earliest drugs to be used effectively in the specific treatment of a particular disease was cinchona bark for malaria. This was introduced in the seventeenth century from Peru and its use was popularized by Sydenham, but it was to be more than one hundred and fifty years, in 1820 to be precise, before quinine was to be isolated from the bark and shown to be the active principle. At this time (and indeed for many more years) the disease for which cinchona was used was the ague.

As cinchona was only effective against malaria, but as the ague was the name applied to any disease accompanied by rigors (uncontrolled shivering), it was not always an effective treatment. This gave different doctors different ideas as to its effectiveness according to whether the patients for whom they had prescribed it had been suffering from genuine malaria or some other disease with rigors. When it is also realized that the correct dosage was not at first known; that the bark was extremely expensive because it came only from Peru, and that because of this charlatans fraudulently sold the bark of cherry trees which had no medicinal value, it will be seen that there were many difficulties to be overcome in establishing it as the genuinely valuable remedy that it was.

It is also worth remarking on the value of cinchona bark in helping to identify malaria. Because cinchona only helped in certain cases of the ague it eventually came to be realized that malaria was a specific disease and that other fevers with rigors had different causes and needed different treatments.

It was, however, more than a century later before the next effective specific drug, digitalis, was to be introduced into medical practice.

In 1785 Dr William Withering in his *An Account of the Foxglove and Some of Its Medical Uses* first introduced the medical profession generally to the therapeutic benefits of digitalis (the leaf of the purple foxglove). He discovered its value after investigating a semi-secret folk medicine in use in Shropshire for dropsy.

> . . . In the year 1775 my opinion was asked concerning a family receipt for the cure of the Dropsy. I was told that it had long been kept a secret by an old woman in Shropshire who had sometimes made cures after the more regular practitioners had failed . . .
>
> . . . The medicine was composed of twenty or more different herbs; but it was not very difficult for one conversant with these subjects to perceive that the active herb could be no other than the Foxglove . . .

The powdered dry leaf was, and still is, very effective in improving the power of the failing heart and thus the circulation. Nowadays the effective principle can be made chemically but the old preparation is still widely used.

During the nineteenth century the ideas and techniques of physics and chemistry were increasingly applied to the problems of medicine and many great strides were made; many substances were isolated in pure form from animal and plant tissues. One of the last chemicals to be discovered in the nineteenth century, in 1899, was acetylsalicylic acid, or aspirin.

However, the real beginning of modern chemotherapy, treatment by means of pure chemicals, dates from Ehrlich's discovery of Salvarsan, compound 606, and its use against syphilis in 1911. Some idea of the magnitude of the work can be guessed from the fact that, not only was it the six hundred and sixth substance made and tested, it was only four years after it was first tested, when *all* the series of substances were re-tested and a mistake discovered, that it possible value was realized.

This number is really quite small by later standards. In a search to find a substitute for quinine, the supplies of which could be cut off in war-time, German chemists made and tested twelve thousand compounds. In Britain, search for a similar drug was only successful on the four thousand, eight hundred and eighty-eighth attempt.

In 1935 came the discovery of prontosil, the first of a class of drugs known as sulphonamides, by Gerhard Domagk. This drug heralded the magnificent progress against infectious disease of the last thirty years. For the first time a substance had been discovered which could be taken in the proper dosage without ill effect but which would prevent the growth of a great variety of germs within the body. Erysipelas and scarlet fever, meningitis and pneumonia could now be treated.

In 1941 came the first publication of the discovery of penicillin. Alexander Fleming's accidental discovery of this in 1928, the later investigations and its eventual production in usable amounts marks a great leap forward in man's struggle against disease.

Penicillin was the first of the antibiotics, the name given to drugs which not only prevent the growth of the germs within the body but actually kill them, and today there are several dozen available. Tuberculosis, for long a major cause of death and disease in early life, is now largely controllable by means of antibiotics. Even cancer in some of its forms can be treated, and in a few of its forms very largely be controlled, by chemotherapeutic measures. There is, however, a long way to go, and the final solution may come from directions quite other than chemotherapy.

In the last few pages we have been mainly concerned with the progress made in discovering drugs which are not normally available to the human being but which can be obtained or made and used to treat disease. These have been mainly drugs used to destroy invading germs or abnormal cells without damaging the healthy tissues of the patient.

There are, of course, other types of disease and one important group is the deficiency diseases. Starvation is a deficiency disease itself but, as the cause and cure are so obvious, it is perhaps hardly considered as a disease although it is a desperately serious condition in many parts of the world today. There is a rather less obvious group of diseases in this class when the deficiency is not so apparent.

In the eighteenth century James Lind, a one-time naval surgeon and later physician to the naval hospital at Haslar, discovered the value of fresh lemon juice and other *fresh* fruits and vegetables in treating and *preventing* scurvy. Other physicians had advised patients suffering from the disease to eat fresh fruit but James Lind was the first to establish it as a proper remedy. In his book *A Treatise on the Scurvy*, 1753, he writes:

> . . . Experience indeed sufficiently shows, that as green or fresh vegetables, with ripe fruits, are the best remedies for it, so they prove the most effectual preservatives against it. And the difficulty of obtaining them at sea, together with a long continuance in the moist sea air, are the true causes of its so general and fatal malignity upon that element . . .

When Lord Anson made the first voyage round the world (1740–1744) he lost seventy-five per cent of his ship's company mainly from scurvy. As a contrast to this, Captain Cook, who followed Lind's advice, on one of his voyages to the Pacific which lasted three-and-a-half years only lost one man from a crew of one hundred and eighteen; and he was ill with consumption before the ship left England. Ships' crews, at sea for months at a time, had previously lived mainly on salt meat and biscuits. After James Lind scurvy became a rare disease in the navy, although it was not until two years after his death that the Board of Admiralty in 1796 officially ordered the use of lemon juice and other fresh fruits and vegetables in ships at sea.

It was not until the twentieth century that scurvy was recognized to be due to lack of Vitamin C in the diet. In 1928 the substance was isolated in a pure form from another source and in 1932 from lemon juice. In 1934, it was synthesized in the laboratory.

It is only in the twentieth century too that it has been realized that there are numerous 'accessory food factors' present in normal diets in small, even minute, quantities which are essential for health. Their absence from the diet causes diseases such as scurvy, beri-beri, pellagra, rickets and others. Many of these have now been discovered and most of them synthesized in the laboratory. These diseases provided that they are treated in time, can now be cured by taking the appropriate vitamins usually in tablet or capsule form. Perhaps more important, they can be prevented by seeing to it that the diet is *not* deficient in any necessary constituents.

The function of vitamins in the body can be looked upon as similar to the oil in a motor car engine. Very little is actually needed and the car will work for a considerable time without fresh supplies but, if it goes on for too long, damage will be done to the engine. If it goes on for just a bit longer, the damage may be too bad to be rectified just by replenishing the oil. The actual quantity used is quite small but that small amount is essential.

During the nineteenth century a great deal of work was done on the ductless glands. These are the glands in the body which make substances, hormones, which are released into the bloodstream and, being transported round the body, then control the workings of many other parts. This work and research into all aspects of nutrition and metabolism, the breaking down and building up of the tissues of the body, has only been possible because of the progress of chemistry.

An example of this is found in the pancreas (sweetbread) which, as well as making digestive juices for the intestines, also makes insulin. This insulin in the blood controls the use of glucose which is a sugar and, if it is insufficient in amount, the patient suffers from diabetes mellitus. The disease of diabetes had been known from ancient times and the fact that the urine of diabetic patients was sweet was recognized in the seventeenth century. It was not, however, until 1889 that the pancreas was definitely incriminated. The crucial investigations, however, to produce insulin were not made until 1921 when insulin was first produced by Banting and Best in Toronto. Before then diabetes could only be controlled at all if mild and then only by severe dieting. Now with proper care, insulin can be administered daily by injection to provide the insulin that the patient is him-

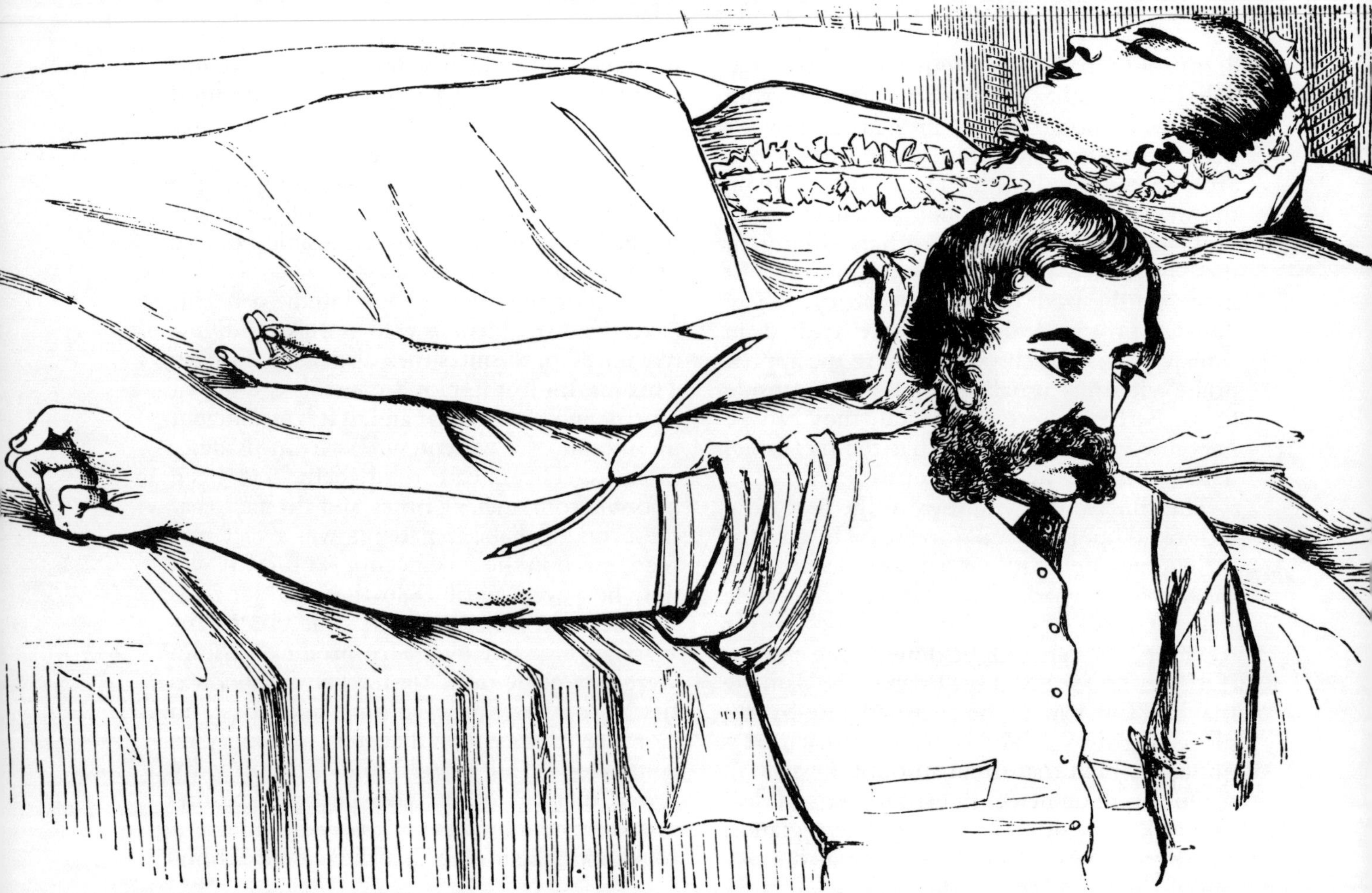

Direct blood transfusion in 1873

self unable to make. The patient can, and usually does, administer this to himself by means of a hypodermic syringe and lead a relatively normal life. Hypodermic syringes for administering drugs beneath the skin have been in use since the middle of the nineteenth century. The one shown below was adapted from other purposes and used by Alexander Wood in about 1855.

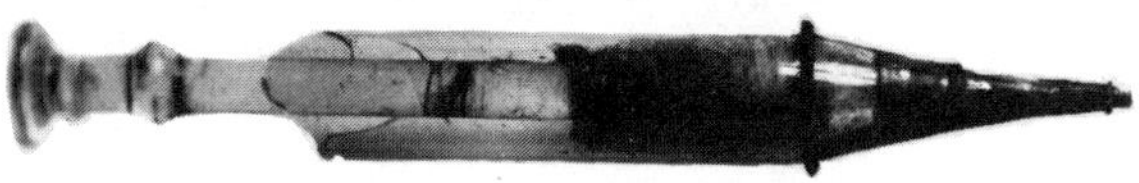

A recent important advance in the field of hormone therapy was the introduction of cortisone in 1949. Cortisone and developments from it have provided medical practitioners with a very powerful drug. It has, however, also many dangers and its eventual place in therapeutics remains to be seen.

Although in the last half-century or so the centre of the therapeutic stage has perhaps been held by chemotherapy, there have been major advances in many other fields.

Blood transfusion is perhaps the greatest of these. Innumerable lives have been saved and many major surgical procedures made possible by the ability to replace blood lost in haemorrhage. Transfusions of blood from animal to animal and from animal to man were made in the seventeenth century, not always with fatal results. But it was not until 1818 that the first transfusion was made from man-to-man. It was, however, the work of Karl Landsteiner in 1900, who showed that all individuals belonged to one of four major different blood groups, that made transfusion a practical reality. Since then many, many less immediately important blood groups have been discovered and matching different bloods is now a highly complicated process. It may be that in time each individual's blood group will be as distinctive as his fingerprint, but it is not always necessary to match all blood groups in transfusions.

In other, perhaps less dramatic but not necessarily less valuable, ways therapy against disease has changed. Nursing (see Chapter Thirteen), physiotherapy, rehabilitation and occupational therapy, dietetics and other forms of help against disease have all developed mainly in the last half-century or less. Space alone prevents consideration of these many changes here.

CHAPTER TWELVE
Epidemic disease and public health

This is from the first account in history by a responsible eyewitness of a major epidemic striking a whole city or country.

> The disease is said to have begun south of Egypt in Ethiopia; . . . For a while physicians sought to apply remedies in ignorance, but it was in vain, and they themselves were most prone to perish because they came into frequent contact with it. No other human art was of any avail . . . so many bodies were lying unburied . . . Some died from want of care but so did others who were receiving the greatest attention . . . But more often the sick and the dying were tended by the pitying care of those who had recovered, . . . For no one was ever attacked a second time, or not with a fatal result . . . Such was the calamity which now afflicted the Athenians . . .

The epidemic occurred in the summer of 430 BC and Thucydides, its author, caught the disease himself but recovered. The nature of the disease is not certain but it may have been the same as is now called Plague (the Black Death of the Middle Ages) which last visited England in 1665 as the Great Plague of London. In September 1665, in one week in London eight thousand, two hundred and ninety-seven persons were *known* to have died, and at that time the population of London was less than one-tenth of what it is to-day. In 1894, one hundred thousand people died from it in Canton in China.

It was not really understood until the nineteenth century that great benefit to a whole nation could be gained by nation-wide measures to protect people from disease. This is not so surprising when one remembers that the knowledge that germs convey disease was discovered only during the nineteenth century.

Measures to protect the health of the general public had indeed been taken in certain instances long before, but only to deal

The Plague of Ashdod by Nicholas Pou

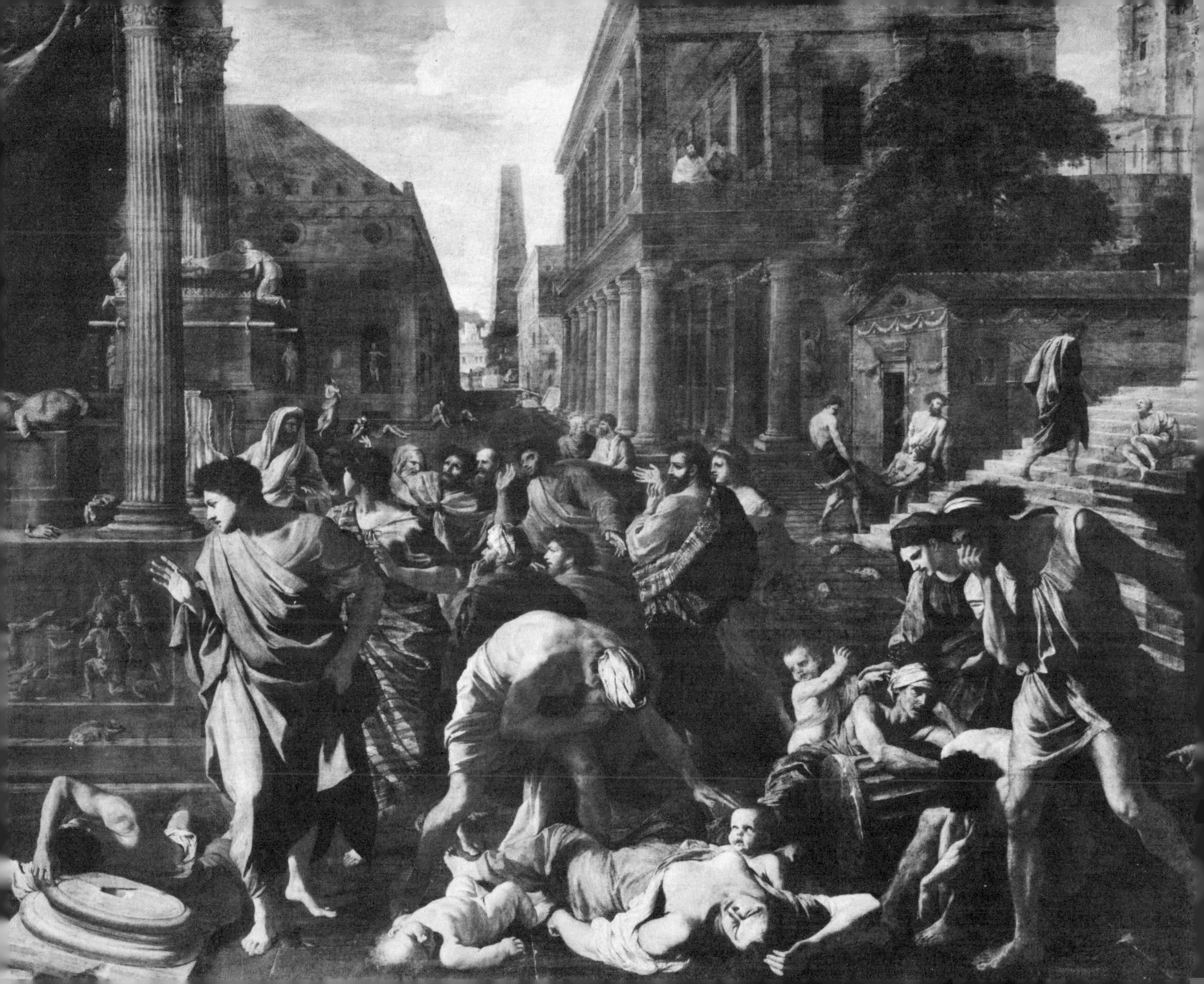

with isolated problems. Leprosy from very ancient times has been regarded as contagious. The Bible directs:

> . . . He shall remain unclean as long as he has the disease; he is unclean; he shall dwell alone in a habitation outside the camp.

Even today leprosy is regarded with somewhat excessive fear. It is not a very infectious ailment but lepers still live in separate settlements in many parts of the world.

Some measures to protect the health of the public were taken in Italy as early as 1377 when ships were isolated and travellers detained at the port for forty days (quaranta giorni – from which the word quarantine comes). Today quarantine for human beings is no longer necessary for travellers entering a country. Much more is known about how disease is spread and preventive measures can be, and are, taken both nationally and internationally against the introduction and spread of infectious disease in a country.

Quarantine measures are still necessary to prevent certain diseases of animals (some of which may also affect man) entering a country. Rabies, or hydrophobia, is a disease of dogs and some other animals: the dog becomes mad and a bite from a rabid dog transmits the disease to the person bitten. The last outbreak in animals in England occurred in 1918–1922, but since then twenty-two cases have developed in quarantine kennels, which shows the value of the quarantine regulations. Misguided dog lovers still sometimes try to smuggle in pet dogs but the regulations are enforced stringently.

Although rabies is still invariably and very horribly fatal once symptoms have developed, it can be prevented due to the magnificent work of Louis Pasteur (see Chapter Eight) if treatment is started soon enough after the bite. The very first occasion on which rabies was effectively treated was in 1885, whilst Pasteur was still conducting his experiments only with animals.

On the morning of July 4th, 1885, Théodore Vone, a grocer of Meissengott, had been attacked by his own dog which had gone mad. Before being caught and killed the dog had savaged a boy, Joseph Meister. This boy, brought by his mother and accompanied by Théodore Vone who had also been bitten, travelled to Paris and in Pasteur's own words:

> . . . three individuals from Alsace unexpectedly presented themselves at my laboratory, on Monday 6th of last July (1885).

Théodore Vone, grocer, . . . bitten in the arm (but because the dog's fangs had not penetrated the skin he was not in danger) . . .

Joseph Meister, aged 9 years, also bitten on July 4th, at eight o'clock in the morning, by the same dog. This child . . . presented numerous bites, on the hands, legs, and thighs, some of them so deep as to render walking difficult . . .

At the examination of the dog, after its death by the hand of its master, the stomach was found full of hay, straw and scraps of wood. The dog was certainly rabid. Joseph Meister had been pulled out from under him covered with foam and blood . . . The death of this child appearing to be inevitable, I decided, not without lively and sore anxiety, as may well be believed, to try upon Joseph Meister the method which I found constantly successful with dogs . . . Consequently, on July 6th, at 8 o'clock in the evening, sixty hours after the bites . . . young Meister was inoculated . . . In the following days fresh inoculations were made. I thus made thirteen inoculations, and prolonged the treatment to ten days. . . . Since the middle of August I have looked forward with confidence to the future good health of Joseph Meister . . .

This first example of laboratory immunology raised resistance to disease by administering artificially weakened germs.

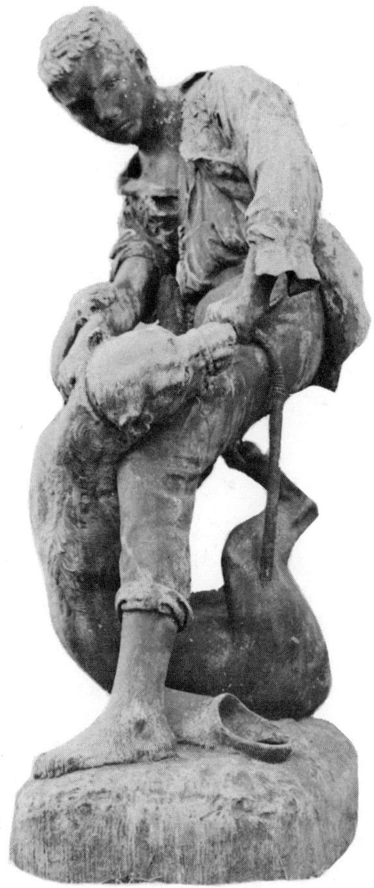

Statue of the lad Jupille, Pasteur's second patient

This was not, however, the first example of artificial immunity. Smallpox from very ancient times has been a major killing disease. Not only did it kill easily but, if the victims recovered, they were usually left scarred for life. Macaulay wrote in his *History of England* concerning Queen Mary who died of smallpox on 28th December 1694.

> ... The havoc of the plague had been far more rapid: but the plague had visited our shores only once or twice within living memory; and the smallpox was always present, filling the churchyards with corpses, tormenting with constant fears all whom it had not yet stricken, leaving on those whose lives it spared the hideous traces of its power ...

There were, as there still are, a major and a minor type of smallpox. The minor type of the disease is much less serious and about ninety-eight per cent of patients who have it recover. There is also much less scarring. In China, at least from the eleventh century, it had been the practice to inoculate people with material obtained from someone with the mild disease with the intention of giving them the mild form of the illness and thereby giving them protection against the more severe form. This practice was introduced to Europe by Lady Mary Wortley Montague, wife of the English ambassador to Turkey, in 1718. It did, however, produce the disease of smallpox and, as such, could be passed on to others. It was not always as mild as was hoped; some people died and some scars were left.

In 1798 Edward Jenner, a country doctor in Gloucestershire, published his investigations concerned with cow-pox (Variolae Vaccinae) which he had begun two years earlier in 1796. Cow-pox was not a very common disease of cows but, when it did occur, the cows developed blisters on the udders and frequently the milkmaids contracted it on their hands. Folklore had it in Gloucestershire that if a dairymaid had once had cow-pox she would not contract smallpox. Jenner proved this to be so and showed how cow-pox could be given to anyone to render them immune to smallpox. A Dorsetshire farmer, Benjamin Jesty, had actually done the same thing with his wife and two children twenty-two years earlier in 1774. This had not been followed up and was almost certainly unknown to Jenner.

Jenner's methods almost immediately received general acceptance and vaccination (as his method was called) was practised

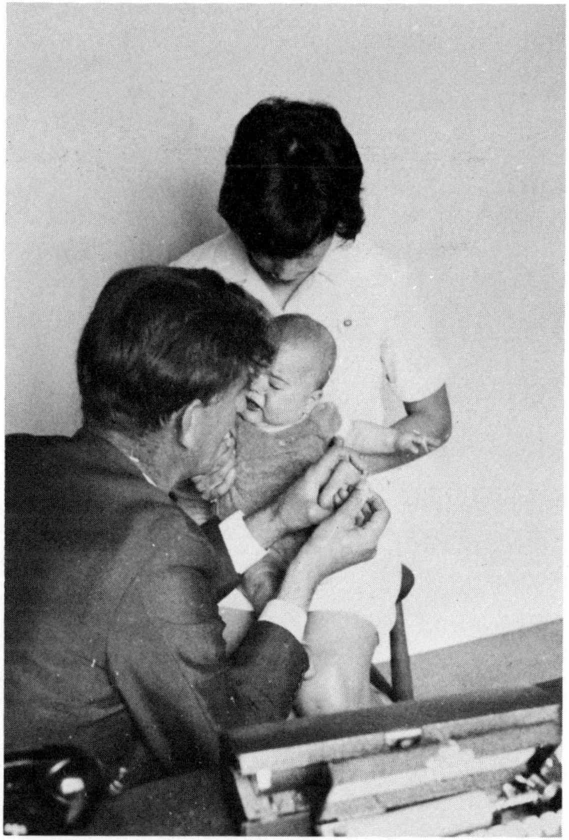

Routine vaccination against smallpox

throughout the world. The first vaccination in America was performed by Dr Waterhouse on his five-year-old son Daniel soon afterwards, in 1800.

Vaccination against smallpox was made compulsory in England by an Act of Parliament passed in 1853, but ninety-five years later in 1948, when the National Health Service Act became law, this was repealed.

A further step in the treatment of infectious disease was the discovery in 1890 – the result of work by many different men – that, if a horse was injected first with killed diphtheria germs and later with live diphtheria germs, the horse had become immune to the disease *and that the serum taken from the horse could be used to treat diphtheria* in humans. The first anti-diphtheria toxin injection, as it was called, was given to a child in Berlin on Christmas night, 1891.

From work of this sort has developed the present practice of infants being immunized as a matter of course in their first few months of life against diseases which, not so long ago, were major killing diseases in every civilized country in the world. In Britain, for instance, it is routine practice now to immunize all infants against diphtheria, whooping cough,

Form of certificate prescribed by the
International Sanitary Regulations
and supplied in the United Kingdom by the
MINISTRY OF HEALTH, LONDON
Scottish Home and Health Department, Edinburgh
Ministry of Health and Social Services, Belfast

INTERNATIONAL CERTIFICATE OF VACCINATION
OR REVACCINATION AGAINST SMALLPOX

CERTIFICAT INTERNATIONAL DE VACCINATION
OU DE REVACCINATION CONTRE LA VARIOLE

This is to certify that
Je soussigné(e) certifie que

FOLD HERE

name ....
nom

date of birth .... sex ....
né(e) le *sexe*

whose signature follows
dont la signature suit

....

has on the date indicated overleaf been vaccinated or revaccinated against smallpox, with a freeze-dried or liquid vaccine certified to fulfil the recommended requirements of the World Health Organization.

a été vacciné(e) ou revacciné(e) contre la variole à la date indiquée au verso, avec un vaccin lyophilisé ou liquide certifié conforme aux normes recommandées par l'Organisation Mondiale de la Santé.

IMPORTANT: See the Rules and Notes on the back.

This certificate, if folded along the central vertical line, can be kept in a passport (with a rubber band).

International vaccination certificate

tetanus, smallpox, poliomyelitis and sometimes measles. Tuberculosis immunization is done usually at a later age.

People travelling to foreign parts, especially the tropics, can be immunized (and in many cases it is a necessity before they can be admitted to certain countries abroad) against many more diseases, particularly yellow fever, cholera, typhoid and paratyphoid fevers. In special cases other immunizations are possible also.

The success that has been achieved in dealing with these diseases has, as explained above, been due partly to preventing and treating the diseases in people, but there is another aspect that is no less important. If the germ causing the disease does not reach the individual, then the individual will not become ill. When the germ passes from person to person as in smallpox, or is injected by means of the bite of a mad dog with rabies, the ideal method of prevention can fairly easily be seen, even if it is not so easy to carry it out.

A great deal of research has been put into discovering how some diseases spread. For a long time malaria was thought to be due to bad air (from the French mal aire) and influenza to 'an influence'. It it now known that particular germs which are carried in particular ways are responsible. Malaria and yellow fever are conveyed by the bite of one kind of mosquito, plague by the bite of a rat flea which lives mainly on black rats, typhus by a body louse, cholera, and sometimes typhoid and paratyphoid by water.

The control of cholera in England provides a good example of how public health measures can sometimes by quite simple means prevent what might otherwise be devastating epidemics. Cholera is a disease due to a germ which is easily carried in water. This disease was unknown in Britain until 1831 when, brought from the Orient, a severe epidemic occurred. Serious epidemics recurred in 1848–1849 and again in 1853–1854 and lesser ones in 1868 and 1893.

Although cholera germs were not actually discovered until 1883 by the German scientist Robert Koch, at the end of the 1848–1849 epidemic John Snow, who was the first anaesthetist in Britain and twice gave anaesthetics to Queen Victoria, had suggested that the disease was due to contamination of water supplies by sewage. He had found that most of the cholera deaths had occurred in an area which obtained its water supply from

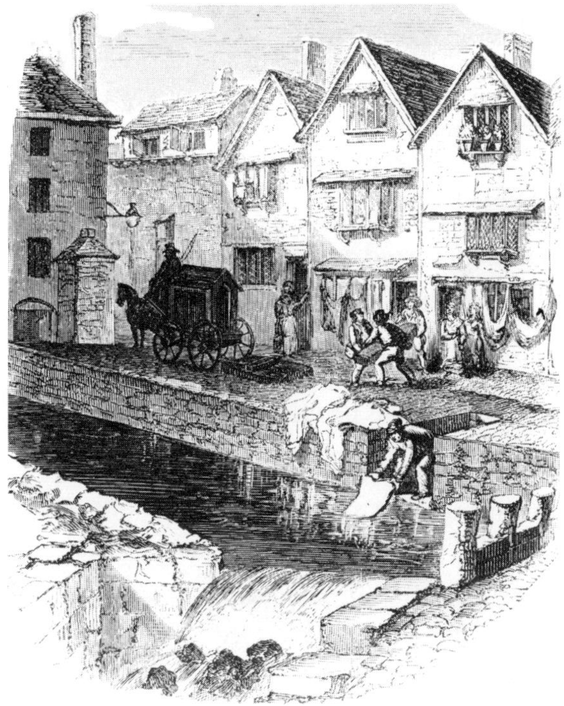

Bed linen from a case of cholera being washed in the stream which supplied Exeter with drinking water during the epidemic of 1832

the River Thames in a place where sewage pollution was especially heavy. This led him to suggest what we now know to be true, that the disease was conveyed by sewage contaminating drinking water.

During the next epidemic in 1854 Snow investigated a small area in London near Golden Square where over five hundred deaths occurred in ten days. He discovered that almost all the houses in which deaths had occurred obtained their water from one pump in Broad Street. He advised that the pump be closed. The pump handle was removed so that people could not get water and the epidemic ceased almost at once, thus providing a lesson in the value of official measures taken to protect public health which has served as an example ever since.

With regard to epidemic and endemic diseases generally, although there are still many, the work that has led to solving many of them has been truly international. Almost all of it has been done during the last century by doctors all over the world, as far apart as Cuba and Japan, America and Italy.

The discovery that Malta fever was due to germs in milk from goats, and that about half the goats on the island of Malta were infected shows how public health measures can alter the incidence of disease. The research that led to the discovery about Malta fever was undertaken by a Commission appointed on behalf of the British armed forces in Malta. When the source of the disease was discovered the armed forces were ordered not to drink unboiled goats' milk. The table opposite demonstrates the dramatic effect this had.

They also point to something else. Whereas rules regarding diet could be enforced in the army and navy, it was much less easy to get the civilian population to comply. It is quite likely that many cases of Malta Fever in the civilian population went unrecorded so that the actual number of cases was higher than those shown in the table.

Until the early part of the nineteenth century, when the problems of epidemic and endemic disease first began to be investigated seriously and scientifically, it had been believed that disease and filth were found together in certain classes of people rather than that disease might be due to filth alone.

But in the early part of the century the idea that disease might be due to filth (rather than germs in filth as the existence of germs was not yet known) began to be considered

Year	In armed forces stationed in Malta	Civilians in Malta
1905	913	663
1906	308	822
1907	21	714
1908	11	502
1909	11	456
1910	4	318

Number of recorded cases of Malta fever

seriously. We have already seen how John Snow regarded cholera as a filth disease and how, without any knowledge of the existence of the cholera vibrio (germ), his methods of preventing filth contamination were effective.

At about the same time as Snow was beginning his investigations Edwin Chadwick, a lawyer not directly connected with medicine, began to play an important part making the nation aware of the need for public health measures and in putting them into practice. He saw the impossibility of individuals themselves being able to do much about it and the great need for governmental – both central and local – action.

He carried out extensive investigations and, in 1842, his *Report on the Sanitary Conditions of the Labouring Population* gave an impetus to public health measures, the benefits of which we are enjoying today.

> . . . with broken panes in every window-frame, and filth and vermin in every nook. With the walls unwhitewashed for years, black with the smoke of foul chimneys, without water, with

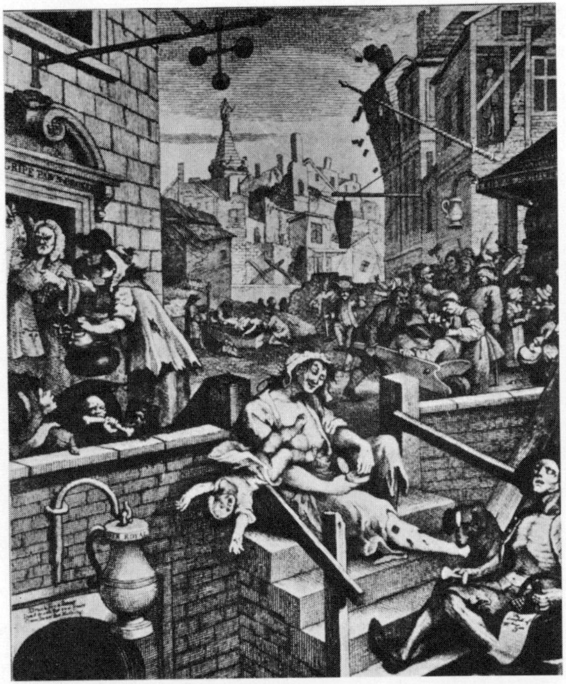

Gin Lane, a satirical drawing by Hogarth, 1751

corded bed-stocks for beds, and sacking for bed clothing, with floors unwashed from year to year, without out-offices [latrines] . . . there are streets, elevated a foot, sometimes two, above the level of the causeway, by the accumulation of years, and stagnant puddles here and there with their foetid exhalations, causeways broken and dangerous, and places choked up with filth, and excrementitious deposits on all sides as a consequence, undrained, unpaved, unventilated, uncared-for . . . Can we wonder that such places are the hot-beds of disease, . . . Adult life, exposed to such miasmata, gives way. How much more then infant life . . .

RECAPITULATION AND CONCLUSIONS

. . . . that the formation of all habits of cleanliness is obstructed by defective supplies of water . . . that the primary and most important measures, and at the same time the most practicable . . . are drainage, the removal of all refuse of habitations, streets and roads, and the improvement of the supplies of water . . .

This work of Chadwick's, together with all the other work that he instigated and undertook between 1832 and 1854, aided and encouraged by Lord Ashley later the Earl of Shaftesbury, led on to the conception of public health that we know today.

Whilst this was going on many other steps, not obviously associated with medicine but which ultimately affected the health of the nation, were taking place in Britain. The Factory Acts of 1833 and 1847 limited the working hours of children and began the inspection and control of safety in places of work, and in 1836 an act provided for the registration of births, marriages and deaths.

The first Medical Officer of Health of any town or city was appointed in Liverpool in 1847 together with an Inspector of Public Nuisances, who was later to be called the Sanitary Inspector and who is now called the Public Health Inspector. The appointment of a Public Health inspector was to lead in time to the appointment of other officials to inspect and control such things as milk and meat supplies.

In London the first Medical Officer of Health was appointed in 1848 and today every part of Britain is under the responsible and watchful eyes of a Medical Officer of Health and his staff.

Towards the close of the century it was realized that a healthy adult population began with healthy children and, in 1890, the London School Board appointed a medical officer to examine children in elementary schools. In 1907 it became compulsory for children to be examined on entering school. Special schools for handicapped children, such as those for the blind and deaf, began in 1908.

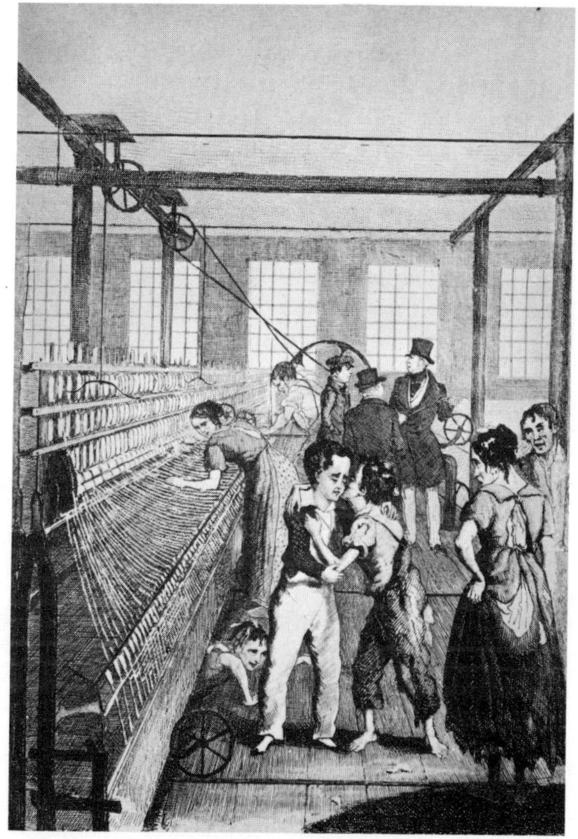

Child labour in textile factories

The realization that health depended not only on cleanliness and freedom from infection but also on adequate nutrition and such things as vitamins (see Chapter Eleven), and that if these things were not provided in early life they could not always be made good in later life, led to free distribution of milk in schools. This began in France in 1894 and in England in 1899. School meals were authorized in 1906.

Going back a step further, it was appreciated that a healthy birth was a desirable beginning to a healthy life. In 1902 the midwives Act made it necessary for all midwives to be properly registered and trained. Whereas in 1899 of every thousand babies born alive one hundred and eighty-nine had died before the age of one year, the rate is now not much over twenty in every thousand.

During the last hundred years a much greater understanding of the problems of health and disease has developed. This has been reflected in medical practice and resulted in enormous changes in the patterns of disease. Whereas a hundred years ago infectious diseases such as diphtheria and tuberculosis were common and frequently fatal, nowadays the first is a very rare disease indeed in Britain and most other countries and the second is becoming infrequent and can be cured by drugs.

On the other hand, diseases of the heart and circulation and cancer in all its forms are both very much more in evidence than they were a hundred years ago. Partly this is due to the greater expectation of life today – more people grow older to suffer from diseases which do not often occur in youth. This is partly due to other factors associated with the changes in the mode of life in the twentieth century. Cigarette smoking is an important factor in causing cancer of the lung; smoke and fumes from the factories and traffic contribute to chronic bronchitis; and the speed and volume of traffic makes road accidents a serious problem. As the conditions under which we live change so do the various diseases assume greater or lesser importance. There are, however, still many of the age old problems to be solved.

A hundred years ago the idea of a whole nation taking action in the cause of health was a new concept. Today, however, there is a World Health Organization. This was established in 1948 with headquarters in Geneva and regional centres for most areas

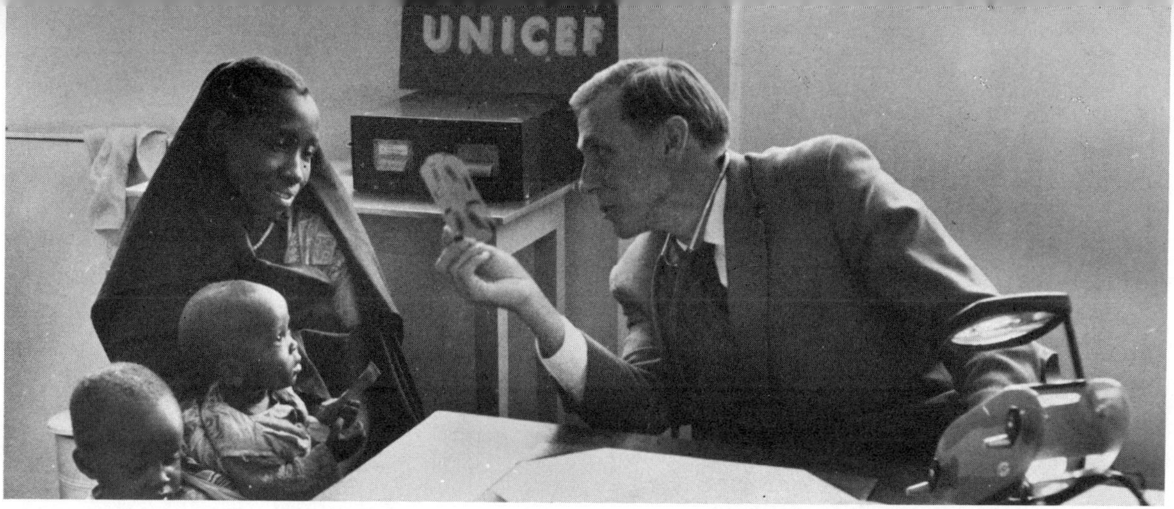

Child welfare is cared for throughout the world by UNICEF

of the world. It is part of the United Nations Organization, as is the United Nations Children's Fund (UNICEF), and both have contributed enormously to world health.

At present there are nearly one hundred nation members of the Organization and it is hoped that one day the entire world will co-operate. The Organization exists to promote all forms of health measures particularly on an international scale. It collects information, produces statistics and organizes conferences. It undertakes various measures on a large scale to try to control certain endemic and epidemic diseases such as yellow fever and malaria. Its most impressive achievements have been in the eradication of the yellow fever mosquito from large areas of South America and malaria from several areas of the world. It assists with emergency aid where this is necessary and has done so in several parts of the world. It assists in education both medical, for which it provides over a thousand fellowships a year, and general health education.

With increasing medical knowledge, changes may occur in the next century as great as those we have been discussing. Whatever these might be the World Health Organization will attempt to play its part. But this is for the future and not yet history.

CHAPTER THIRTEEN
The practice of medicine

We do not know much of the ordinary practitioner of Ancient Egypt but such there must have been. When, some five thousand years or so ago, an ordinary Egyptian developed a pain or injured a limb, it is unlikely that he would have had the benefit of being treated by an eminent physician such as Imhotep.

There does, however, seem little doubt that, from a very early date, there were not only medical specialists but also specialized helpers such as nurses, masseurs and bandagists. There is even evidence of a sort of state-controlled medical service. There were physicians, physician inspectors, chief physicians, a Chief Physician of the North and South, a Court Physician, a Chief of Physicians of the Palace, a Chief Physician of the King. As some, and perhaps all, of these were paid by the state, it does at least seem possible that the Egyptian workman had the benefit of something similar to a National Health Service!

How medical education was obtained is not clear but it was probably through the apprenticeship system. That is to say, the pupil worked with an experienced physician who taught him all that he knew. This was probably combined with attendance at a House of Life. Since at this time physicians had to follow accepted medical practice, with considerable penalties if they did not and the patient died, there must have been some state control to see that the practice was enforced.

Some women physicians also practised but evidence so far does not point to many and, with the exception of the ladies of Salerno, who might have been physicians, midwives or nurses, women physicians do not appear again until the nineteenth century. There are references to midwives in Rome and remedies being provided by women, but these ladies were not likely to have been physicians so much as users of home remedies.

In Greece and Rome the physician seems to have been highly esteemed. His training was again mainly through the apprenticeship system, but those who could afford the time and expense involved perhaps journeyed to centres of medical learning, of which, until the first century BC, Alexandria was the chief one, and spent some time there. There was no recognized qualification but probably the best jobs were more readily available to those who could prove that they had studied diligently at Alexandria. In the first century BC a Greek, Asclepiades of Bithynia, founded a medical school in Rome. It continued after his death and others developed. There is also some evidence of Roman medical schools in other places in the Empire, perhaps for the training of army surgeons. In the first century AD some medical teachers were paid by the state and lecture halls were provided for the teaching of medicine. We have already seen in Chapter Three how the writings of Celsus and, in the second century AD, Galen, influenced medical thought.

Except for the Arabian physicians, after the Romans medical knowledge, in so far as there was any, was largely confined to the monks. Few other people could read what books there were. Then came the establishment of a medical centre at Salerno followed by the establishment of centres of medical learning in Northern Italy and at Montpellier, as we have already seen in Chapter Four.

During the Middle Ages and the early years of the Renaissance in Europe barber-surgeons developed alongside the physicians and apothecaries. As barbers had sharp instruments for trimming beards and cutting tonsures, it is not perhaps surprising that they should have been asked to cut for blood. There were also wandering craftsmen or surgeons who specialized in 'cutting for the stone' and some who operated on the eyes for cataracts. All these surgeons were practical men who plied a trade often enough without learning and without respect for the academic and not very practical learning of the physicians. The physicians in turn had little regard for the uncouth, unlettered and untaught surgeons.

There were also the apothecaries. These were men who collected, stored and sold drugs and remedies. Although in the beginning they were not directly connected with medicine at all, being associated with spicers and pepperers or grocers, they gradually became a distinct trade providing drugs and

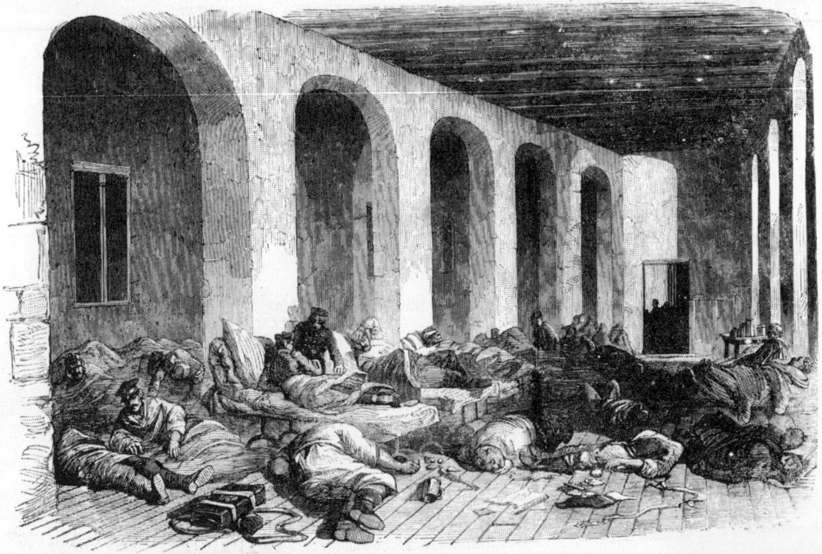

A ward in a hospital at Sebastapol before the arrival of Florence Nightingale in the Crimea

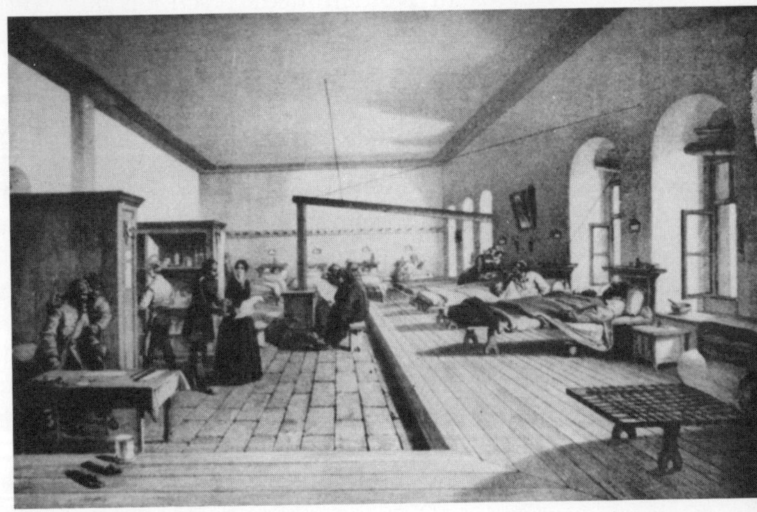

Florence Nightingale in the hospital at Scutari; the changes that she brought about are evident by comparison with the picture above

medicaments on the prescriptions of the physicians. Naturally enough, their advice was sought by patients as to what remedy was required until gradually they became more physician-dispensers than grocer-salesmen. As the physicians of this time were relatively few in numbers, the apothecaries, with their direct contacts with people, gained from practical experience what they lacked in academic learning. There were also wandering pedlars of various herbs and drugs including probably many charlatans.

Because all these various types of men were associated with medical practice in one way or another there were many jealousies and disagreements. However, during the sixteenth century in Britain, the various practitioners began to straighten out their differences and to realize the need for better organization of their various professions and trades. It came to be appreciated that, both to protect the patients from glib-tongued but unqualified men and to advance the study of medicine and surgery, there needed to be some form of central association and control.

The first of these central governing bodies in Britain was the Incorporation of Barber Surgeons in Edinburgh granted in 1505 by the Town Council of Edinburgh and confirmed in 1506 by King James IV. This body became the Royal College of Surgeons of Edinburgh in 1778 as it is to the present day. In 1599 the Faculty of Physicians and Surgeons in Glasgow was formed. In England an Act of Parliament was passed in 1511 requiring physicians and surgeons to be licensed by the Bishop of London or Dean of St Paul's, but in 1518 this was effectively (though the law was not actually repealed until 1948) replaced by King Henry VIII granting under the Great Seal letters patent incorporating the President and College or Commonalty of the Faculty of Medicine of London. In 1551 it became The Royal College of Physicians of London. It was empowered to examine and license practitioners and to decide who should practise in the City of London and within a radius of seven miles of it. Henry VIII also gave the royal assent to a union between the guilds of barber-surgeons and surgeons in 1540. This established that surgeons should no longer be barbers and that barbers should restrict their surgery to dentistry.

It was not, however, until 1858, three years after a Medical Register had been compiled, that the General Medical Council was formed with power to decide what qualifications were necessary for a practitioner to be included in the register. This, of course, meant that the General Medical Council would control medical education. Any university (or for that matter any other body) could give whatever medical education it chose, but the General Medical Council would not recognize the degree or diploma for inclusion in the Medical Register unless it approved of the training. It is, however, still possible for a person to practise as a physician or indeed a surgeon without being on the Medical Register. There are many bonesetters and unorthodox practitioners in practice today who are not registered by the General Medical Council, and not by any means all are charlatans. They cannot, however, perform certain functions. They cannot, for instance, sign death certificates, attend at confinements as doctors or prescribe certain drugs. They cannot be employed in the National Health Service as doctors.

This control over the education and training of medical practitioners by the General Medical Council ensures that the public (the patients) cannot be deluded by charlatans and ensures high standards of practice and of general behaviour. Medical practitioners can be struck off the register if they are guilty of offences such as drunkenness or addiction to drugs or improperly associating with patients.

This control of training and qualification has extended to many of the professions associated with medicine. The Professions Supplementary to Medicine Act of 1960 marked a further step in this direction by providing for state registration in such professions as those of Physiotherapy, Radiography, Chiropody and Medical Laboratory Technology.

Nursing can perhaps be said to be older than medical practice itself as a means of helping one's fellow beings. As a profession it is not easy to say where or when it began. New Zealand was the first country to establish State Registration of Nursing in 1901 followed rapidly by some American States. It was not, however, until 1919 that it occurred in Britain.

From mediaeval times there have been religious nursing orders. The order of St Francis of Assisi, established in the thirteenth century, was one. The Sisters of Charity of the order of St Vincent de Paul, established in 1634, is another and is now the largest Roman Catholic nursing order in the world.

Nursing in the continent of Europe was usually in advance of that in England until Florence Nightingale's work in the nineteenth century. Until her time there was no sort of qualification or training for nursing other than that given by religious orders. Nursing was generally regarded as, and generally was, a menial task combining domestic duties in the wards with some attention to patients. When Guy's Hospital in London was opened in 1725 the *Daily Post* commented that higher rates of pay were given to prevent the nurses and other servants from extorting money from the patients. In 1726 the minutes of the Court of Committees of Guy's show that embezzling provisions, pawning patients' clothes, drunkenness, admitting disorderly people and neglect of patients were frequent occurrences.

Florence Nightingale herself came from a wealthy family and her desire to enter nursing was looked upon at first as ridiculous and impossible. She herself wrote:

> The thoughts and feelings that I have now I can remember since I was six years old. . . . The first thought I can remember, and the last, was nursing work; . . .

She attempted to enter nursing at Salisbury Hospital but, although twenty-five years old, she was prevented by her family.

She travelled extensively on the continent of Europe with her family and visited many hospitals. In 1850 she visited a small hospital at Kaiserwerth in Germany where she saw the work that was being done by the Kaiserwerth Deaconesses. These Deaconesses did both the nursing and the domestic work of the hospital in rotation. In 1851 Florence Nightingale, now aged thirty-one, overcame the family's objections and herself went for three months' training at Kaiserwerth. Two years later, in 1853 in London, she opened an Establishment for Gentlewomen during Illness. She was determined to attract a different type of woman into nursing and her real ambition was to train nurses.

Her ideas were just beginning to be appreciated, and she had actually accepted a post as Superintendent of Nurses at King's College Hospital, when the Crimean War broke out in 1854. Instead of going to King's College Hospital she was asked to take a group of nurses to the Crimea and she personally selected a group of eighteen Roman Catholic and Anglican nursing sisters and twenty others from various London hospitals. In the Crimea she was horrified at what she found. The usual conditions can be judged from the first illustration on page ninety-seven. Her first request is said to have been for three hundred scrubbing brushes. Very many lives were saved by her organization of the hospitals and her improvement of the conditions in them. She went round the wards (about four miles of beds) often at night with a lamp to see what was needed for the next day and because of this has become known as 'The Lady of The Lamp'. This was the first time that women had worked in the army and the enormous improvement in hospital conditions can be judged from the second illustration.

On her return to England she set about organizing the training of nurses and, in 1860, The Nightingale School of Nursing was opened at St Thomas' Hospital in London. She was determined to make nursing a proper career for women. How well she succeeded is best judged by the high nursing standards found in almost all hospitals in Britain and most of the rest of the world today.

Perhaps if there had been women doctors in the medical profession this would have occurred earlier, for indeed attention to domestic and personal comforts, which are an important part of nursing, were, in the nineteenth century at least, a field for feminine rather than masculine concern. It was, however, only in the later part of the century that women were accepted as practitioners into the medical profession at all.

The first woman in modern times to qualify as a doctor was Elizabeth Blackwell in New York in 1849. It was not for another sixteen years that a woman was allowed to qualify in Britain. Elizabeth Garrett, later Elizabeth Garrett Anderson, was awarded the diploma of The Society of Apothecaries in 1865 and it was largely as the result of her efforts, and those of Sophia Jex-Blake, that women were gradually accepted into the profession. The story of their struggles to gain recognition for the place of women in medicine is a story of determination and courage in itself.

Edinburgh University was the first British university to admit women medical students in 1869 but they were segregated from the male students and denied many of the facilities of the university. The first five women students admitted, because they were segregated and had to have lectures arranged for the five of them alone, had to pay fees which made it worthwhile for the professors to lecture to them. This made the expense some four times as great as it was for men.

Edith Pechey, one of these five, as a first-year student came first in an examination for a chemistry prize but, because she was a woman, was passed over in favour of a male student who was second on the list.

Sophia Jex-Blake, another of these five, was involved in a libel action as the result of a riot outside Surgeons' Hall. Although judgement in the case went against her, the damages awarded were only one farthing which perhaps indicated the public support for their cause.

In Edinburgh a 'Committee to Secure a Complete Medical Education for Women in Edinburgh' was formed but despite this in 1874, before they had actually qualified, the university expelled them all on the grounds that it had exceeded its authority in admitting them in the first place.

Although they must have been discouraged they did not despair and in 1877 both Edith Pechey and Sophia Jex-Blake qualified as Doctors of Medicine (M.D.) at the University of Berne in Switzerland.

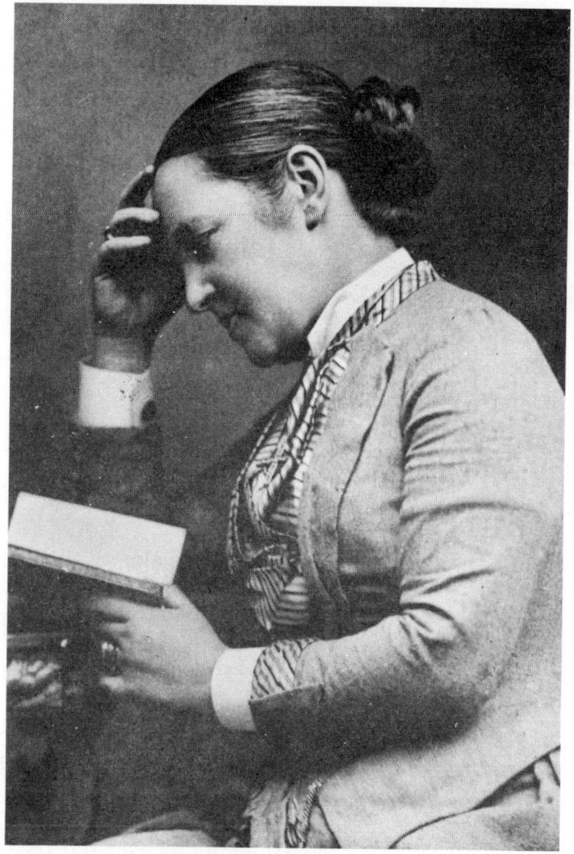

Elizabeth Garrett Anderson

The London School of Medicine for Women was founded, largely as a result of the efforts of Elizabeth Garrett and Sophia Jex-Blake, in 1874 and the inaugural address was given in October, 1877, by Dr Edith Pechey. From then onwards, although facing many difficulties, women have been increasingly accepted into the profession.

In any modern hospital today the work that is done is dependent on the skill and devotion to their work of the doctors, the nurses and the innumerable others involved in the modern hospital. No longer is any branch of medicine closed to either sex and male nurses and women doctors work side by side in the welfare of the patients.

The modern hospital is, of course, a very different place from the hospital of the past. We have already encountered the hospitals of India and Ceylon of more than two thousand years ago and the possibility of hospitals in Egypt even two thousand years earlier than that. 'Arabic' hospitals in Spain and the hospitals for Roman soldiers have also been mentioned. There were also often hospitals or hospital wings attached to monasteries in the Middle Ages, and these were the only hospitals then in existence.

These hospitals were, of course, very different from the modern conception of a hospital. We do not know much detail and it may well be that many of the hospitals were little more than a roof and food for those unable to fend for themselves. Some, however, certainly had physicians regularly attending and if, indeed, the Houses of Life of Ancient Egypt were hospitals than they were probably part of the highest places of learning in the land.

In Britain we know little about the practice of medicine in the very distant past, and not even much about what happened during the time of Roman occupation. In the earliest written history of England, the Venerable Bede wrote:

> ... there was the house to which those who were sick and like shortly to die were carried ...

Throughout the dark and middle ages it is likely that there were hospitals, perhaps often temporary, at times of epidemics.

The earliest hospital founded in England which still exists is St Bartholomew's in London. It was founded about 1123 by the monk Rahere, and is now a famous teaching hospital. St Thomas' Hospital, although not now on its original site, was founded early in the next century. It was not until the eighteenth century that hospitals of a permanent and considerable size began to be built in London and some of the larger towns.

In the early part of the nineteenth century hospitals for special diseases or diseases of particular systems, such as the central nervous system, began to appear. The London Dispensary for Curing Diseases of the Eye and Ears which was founded in 1805 and which later became the Royal Ophthalmic Hospital (better known as Moorfields) is an early example.

From the middle of the nineteenth century cottage hospitals, which were usually hospitals established in villages or small towns, often literally in cottages, began to develop in large numbers. In 1859 Cranleigh Hospital, which was one of the first, was opened and by the end of the century there were over three hundred throughout Britain.

In the latter part of the century, dispensaries which were really 'out-patient' hospitals for the poor and needy began to appear and in time many of these developed into what were known as voluntary hospitals. The voluntary hospitals, which, until the beginning of the National Health Service in 1948 (see below) were an important part of the hospital services of Britain, were hospitals supported largely by private charity. The other type of hospital, known as municipal hospitals, were those hospitals supported by local authorities and often developed from Poor Law Institutions.

The development of the hospitals was the result of many factors but perhaps, from the middle of the nineteenth century onwards, the use of anaesthetics, with the resultant increase in surgery, was one of the most important. When surgery began to be performed for less than desperate reasons there were great advantages in having a centre rather than operating in bedrooms and kitchens. Today the great majority of the functions of a hospital could not be performed away from the complex structure of people and equipment that is the modern hospital.

In 1948, when the National Health Service came into being in Britain, the Government assumed responsibility for some two thousand eight hundred hospitals in England and Wales (excluding Scotland) with approximately five hundred thousand beds. Because of reorganization some beds were closed and in 1949 in

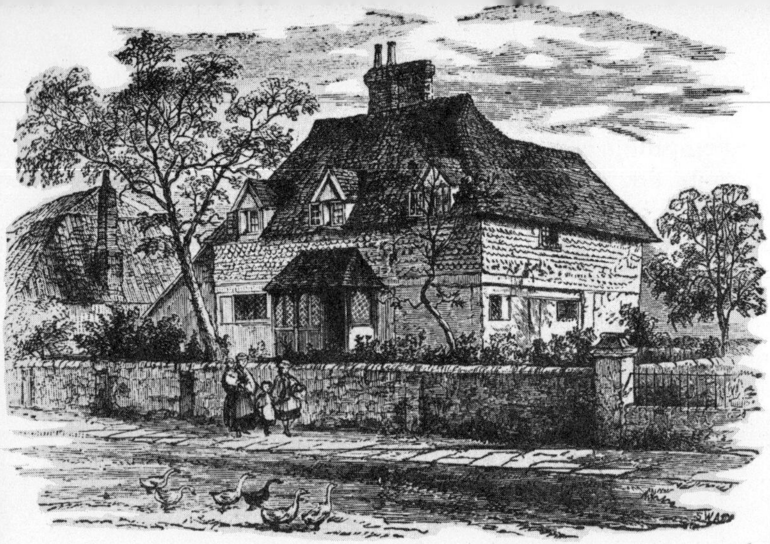

The original building of Cranleigh Village Hospital, opened in 1859 with six beds

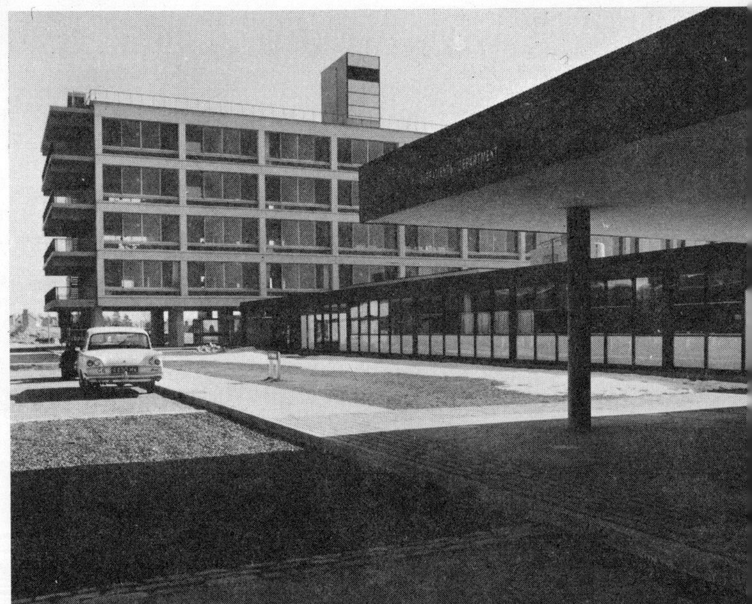

A view of part of the Princess Margaret Hospital, Swindon: present day hospitals have to be designed on a much larger scale.

the National Health Service hospitals in England and Wales there were 475,418 staffed beds. Almost three million in-patients and thirty-six million out-patients and casualties were treated. In 1960 over four million in-patients were treated and over forty-one million out-patients and casualties.

The whole pattern of hospitals in Britain is at present under review and there are plans for great changes and developments. These plans are but one aspect of a great change that has come over medical practice in the middle years of the twentieth century with the great increase in the application of science and technology to medical practice.

We have seen something of how, gradually, especially during the nineteenth century, the state has assumed responsibility for matters of public health. In the twentieth century this has grown into the state accepting an increasing responsibility for matters of personal health. This has occurred in most of the civilized countries of the world but in a variety of different ways. In Britain this has led to a National Health Service which is free at the time of need.

The idea behind free medical treatment is not that medical treatment any more than any other service can be free but that its cost shall be spread over the whole community according to their ability to pay for it. It is, moreover, to be paid for throughout life and not only at times of illness.

In the eighteenth century at least, there were certain compulsory deductions from the pay of seamen both in the British Royal Navy and the American Merchant Navy to provide them with free hospital facilities of a limited sort when they needed them. In Germany, in 1883, an Insurance Act was passed which provided certain health benefits to people when they were ill. Many European nations followed this idea and in Britain, in 1911, an act was passed making it compulsory for a sum of money to be deducted from all workers each week (fourpence from men, threepence from women) to which the employers (threepence) and the Government (twopence) added contributions. These sums of money were to provide a central fund from which payments would be made for medical treatment and sick pay. This scheme provided benefits for the working population but not for wives, children and some others.

In 1941, the Government set up a committee under the chairmanship of Sir William

Beveridge to examine the existing national schemes of social insurance and allied services and to make recommendations for the future. It presented its findings together with its recommendations in a book, *Social Insurance and Allied Services*, better known as *The Beveridge Report*. This formed the basis on which the present social security services in Britain are founded. As regards medicine, it led to the passage of the National Health Service Act, 1946. This led to the formation of the National Health Service, which has already been mentioned, and which came into operation on 5th July 1948.

Since 5th July 1948, as a result of this and other Acts of Parliament, all medical treatment in Britain has been available for everyone in Britain without any direct charge except for small charges which have sometimes been made for prescriptions, and slightly larger ones for some things such as dentures and glasses.

People do not have to take advantage of the National Health Service (the N.H.S.) but everyone has to pay for it by means of taxation. In practice almost all the doctors in Britain are connected with the N.H.S. and very many of them do most or all of their work for it. Patients can, however, still go to a doctor privately, if they wish. This means that they have to pay the doctor for his treatment and for the cost of drugs and medicines as well. They still, however, are obliged to pay their share of the cost of the National Health Service through insurance contributions and general taxation even if they make no use of it at all.

In other countries different methods of insurance have been adopted. In most advanced countries in the world there are now large-scale insurance schemes for medical treatment, often but not always controlled to some extent by the Government of that country. As a result, medical treatment has become much more available to people in need of it often without having to consider the cost. This has brought enormous benefits to many millions of people although it has also made it difficult to appreciate the value of medical services. This has led both to unnecessary usage with consequent waste and also sometimes to unrealistic fears of private costs.

So far, all these health services are in their infancy. There is inherent in most of them the risk to progress that comes with too much central control and too little freedom for individual progress. This is a risk of which many medical practitioners and others are aware and it is to be hoped that controls imposed for the benefit of today will not impede progress for the future.

Just as the magic and mysticism of ancient times needed Hippocrates and his followers to shake medical practice free of wrong ideas: just as the medicine of the Middle Ages needed Vesalius and Harvey to shake off the mistaken ideas of over a thousand years: so also will the ideas of today need revision and rejuvenation.

Such changes are for the future and are not yet history. History, however, plays its part in showing that when men have felt sure of themselves, sure that they knew the truth, something has come along to show that they had not reached the stage of ultimate wisdom. Where progress lies ahead cannot be foretold; it must grow and develop as man grows and develops.

Medicine has always been concerned with the happiness of man. Kindness, consideration, compassion, care: all these are of the essence of medical practice. The great scientific advances of recent years must not obscure the central problem – that of man.

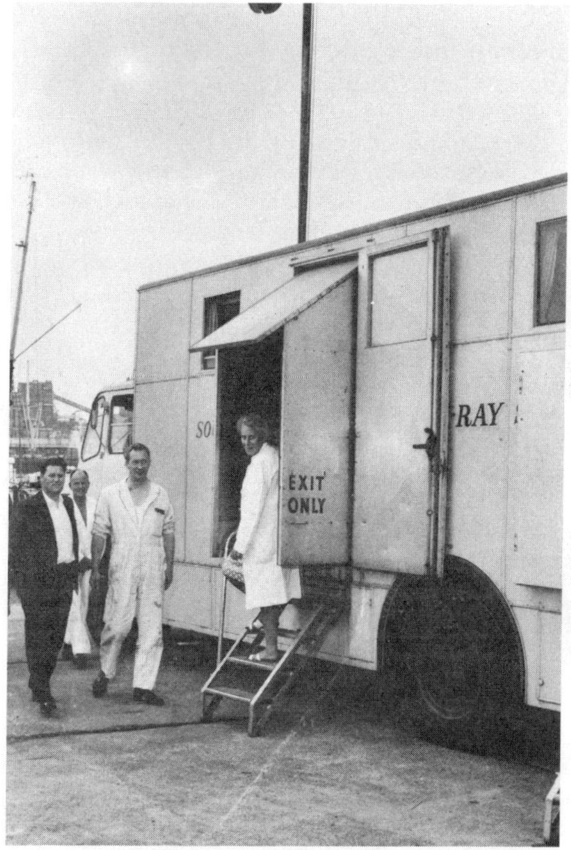

A travelling unit X-rays people at work.

Pope Paul VI in his Coronation speech, speaking not particularly of medicine but of the modern world, said:

> . . . Man of to-day aware of the progress of science and technology, inebriated with successes in fields hitherto unexplored, seems to have deified his own power and to want to surpass God . . .

Great steps in science do indeed tend to blind one to the need still to seek further for the deeper and deeper truth than man is trying to perceive. Sometimes medicine has been subjected to considerable temptations of this sort. It is to be hoped that there will never come a time when any history of medicine can be written without the truth of words from the Hippocratic Collection being as applicable then as they have always been. For 'where there is the love of man, there also is love of the art'.

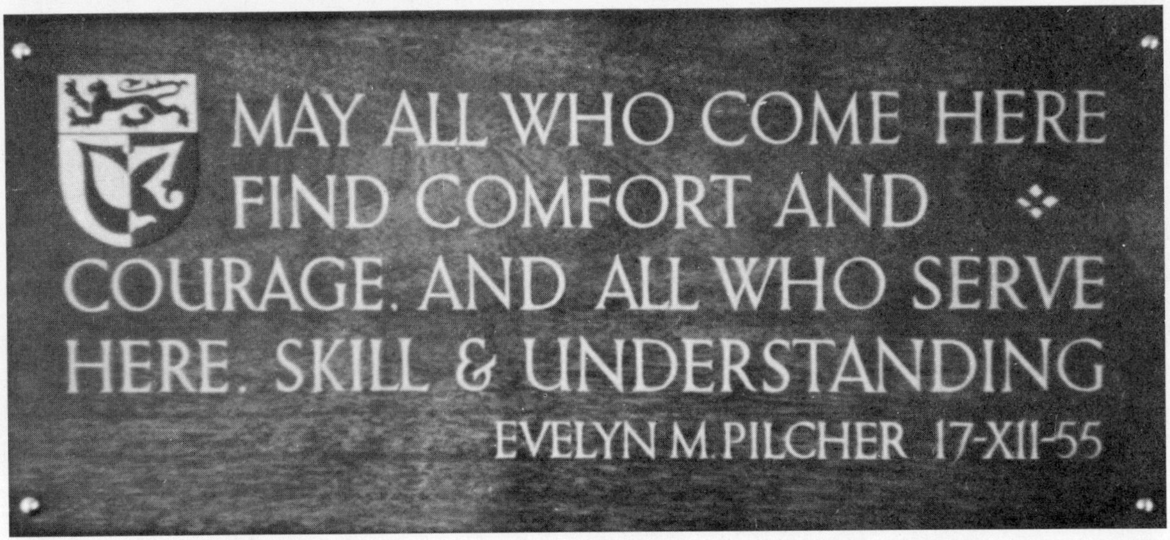

FURTHER INFORMATION

A book of this size can do no more than indicate the broad outlines of the history of medicine over the ages and, in a few places, point to some of the more significant events and people influencing that story.

For those who wish to enquire further into this fascinating field of history there are associations and societies in many parts of the world devoted to the history of medicine and allied subjects. In Britain the Wellcome Institute of the History of Medicine, 183 Euston Road, London, N.W.1., is the foremost centre. Its Museum frequently organizes special exhibitions on particular subjects, and it is the home of the British Society for the History of Medicine which publishes a quarterly journal, *Medical History*.

The following books, which should be obtainable through the Public Library Service, will provide a more detailed glimpse into the subject. The author is indebted to them all:

A Short History of Medicine (760 pages, illustrated), by C. Singer and E. A. Underwood; Oxford University Press, 1962. Despite its title it is an authoritative and fairly comprehensive history.

A History of Medicine (420 pages, illustrated), by D. Guthrie; Nelson and Sons, 1958. This is readable and reliable and is one of the best short general histories.

A Source Book of Medical History (675 pages), edited by L. Clendening; Dover Publications Inc., New York. This is a collection of extracts from original medical literature from the earliest days to the end of the nineteenth century with notes by the compiler-editor.

Science and Secrets of Early Medicine (310 pages with 378 illustrations), by J. Thorwald; Thames and Hudson, 1963. This book deals exclusively with the ancient civilization, although in time this extends to the fourteenth century in the Americas. It is liberally illustrated and simply written.

The Early History of Surgery (186 pages, illustrated), by W. J. Bishop; Robert Hale Ltd., 1960.

World Health and History (243 pages, illustrated), by N. Hobson; John Wright and Sons, 1963.

A Short History of Public Health (210 pages), by C. F. Brockington; J. and A. Churchill Ltd., 1966, is an account of public health measures, mainly in Britain in the nineteenth and twentieth centuries.

The Healers – The Doctor Then and Now (237 pages, illustrated), by K. Pollack and E. A. Underwood; Nelson and Sons, 1968. This book is more about how doctors lived and practised than about 'medicine'.

INDEX